BETTER HEALTH IN HARDER TIMES

Active citizens and innovation on the frontline

Edited by Celia Davies, Ray Flux, Mike Hales and
Jan Walmsley

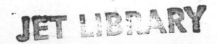

First published in Great Britain in 2013 by

The Policy Press
University of Bristol
Fourth Floor
Beacon House
Queen's Road
Bristol BS8 1QU
UK
Tel +44 (0)117 331 4054
Fax +44 (0)117 331 4093
e-mail tpp-info@bristol.ac.uk
www.policypress.co.uk

North American office:
The Policy Press
c/o The University of Chicago Press
1427 East 60th Street
Chicago, IL 60637, USA
t: +1 773 702 7700
f: +1 773-702-9756
e:sales@press.uchicago.edu
www.press.uchicago.edu

© The Policy Press 2013

British Library Cataloguing in Publication Data
A catalogue record for this book is available from the British Library.

Library of Congress Cataloging-in-Publication Data
A catalog record for this book has been requested.

ISBN 978 1 44730 693 1 paperback
ISBN 978 1 44730 694 8 hardcover

The right of Celia Davies, Ray Flux, Mike Hales and Jan Walmsley to be identified as editors of this work has been asserted by them in accordance with the 1988 Copyright, Designs and Patents Act.

The statements and opinions contained within this publication are solely those of the editors and contributors and not of The University of Bristol or The Policy Press. The University of Bristol and The Policy Press disclaim responsibility for any injury to persons or property resulting from any material published in this publication.

The Policy Press works to counter discrimination on grounds of gender, race, disability, age and sexuality.

Cover design by The Policy Press
Front cover: images kindly supplied by Ray Flux
Printed and bound in Great Britain by Hobbs, Southampton
The Policy Press uses environmentally responsible print partners

FSC
www.fsc.org
MIX
Paper from
responsible sources
FSC® C020438

To Bob Sang (1948–2009), advocate, compulsive networker, facilitator, convivial commuter, social entrepreneur, from friends, for the future; and to Lisa Sang and their children and grandchildren, who remember him far more than we do.

Contents

Contents

Contributors' biographical notes

Kate Ansell is a patient representative at a local and national level and chairman of the Shropshire Patients' Group. She originally worked in town planning, which led to the setting up of the Ironbridge Gorge Museum Trust, and later established an outside catering business employing 50 staff.

Neil Bacon is an entrepreneur and former nephrologist, founder of Doctors.net.uk and owner of the ratings site, www.iWantGreatCare.org.

Yvonne Bennett is a patient with online access to her medical records and secretary of the patient participation group of her GP practice. She is involved in promoting online access to medical records, through articles and presentations.

Laurie Bryant is a graduate and is supported by mental health services. He has worked nationally and internationally in developing improved services. He has found that genuine partnership was always a prerequisite to any success.

Nan Carle is a passionate and seasoned advocate for inclusive communities. She has successfully challenged and changed policy and practice to give communities in several different countries the skills and knowledge to resolve conflicts effectively and unleash the power of individuals to manage well and live fully, at work and at home.

Rohhss Chapman has worked in partnership with learning-disabled people since 1990 and is a lecturer in learning disability studies at the University of Manchester. She supported Carlisle People First (now People First Independent Advocacy) to set up their own self-advocacy company.

Tim Craft is medical director at the Royal United Hospital in Bath and leads continuous improvement programmes that weave together safety, patients' experiential feedback and clinical outcome data.

Georgina Craig is a member of the NHS Alliance executive, leading on pharmacy commissioning and co-leading on the Alliance's patient and public involvement network. In 2011, she completed a Department of Health-funded pilot of 'Experience-Led Commissioning' (ELC) and is now working to spread ELC across the NHS and build its evidence base.

Ian Cunningham has worked with organisations on organisation-wide change, with Boards on strategy development, with teams on their development, and through individual mentoring and coaching of Chief Executive Officers and other senior leaders. He has created innovative development programmes for more than 40 organisations.

Catherine Dale is programme manager for patient-centred care in King's Health Partners Integrated Cancer Centre. She has 12 years' experience managing in acute trusts, has set up a PALS service and developed the King's Fund's online Experience-Based Co-Design toolkit.

Celia Davies is a sociologist with a long-standing interest in research on and with the health professions, and Professor Emerita of Health Care at The Open University. She carried out a pioneering small study of lay members on health professional regulatory bodies in 2000 and is a lay member of the General Pharmaceutical Council.

Simon Duffy is director of The Centre for Welfare Reform, an honorary research fellow at the University of Birmingham and policy advisor to the Campaign for a Fair Society. He was an early pioneer of supported living, person-centred planning, self-directed support and citizenship-focused public policy. He has a doctorate in moral philosophy.

Simon Eaton is a consultant physician and diabetologist in Northumbria Healthcare NHS Foundation Trust based at North Tyneside General Hospital and clinical lead for long-term conditions for NHS North East. He leads a programme to drive transformational change and quality improvements in services, to improve outcomes for people with long-term conditions. Simon was a Health Foundation Leadership Fellow in 2007–09.

Brian Fisher is a semi-retired GP and a founder-director of PAERS Ltd (Patient Access to Electronic Record Systems). He is active in patient and public involvement in the primary care sector in Lewisham and in the NHS Alliance, and is a fellow of the Centre for Welfare Reform.

Angela Flux has been a teacher focusing on religious, personal and social education, an adult educator in health issues, and a pioneer in adolescent peer education, particularly in sexual health. She has worked on the interface between local government and community groups, designing and managing health and well-being programmes at local level.

Ray Flux has worked for more than 20 years as an independent consultant on the interface between clinical professions and services and the people who use or work alongside them. Before that, he was a fellow at the King's Fund. He works to develop partnerships and dialogue in health economies at local and regional levels.

Catherine Foot is a senior fellow in policy at the King's Fund, focusing on aspects of quality. Previously, she was head of policy at Cancer Research UK and she has helped to lead a number of voluntary sector coalitions.

Beryl Furr has worked with many individual patients and communities of interest, in roles that include non-executive director in a Primary Care Trust, chief officer of a community health council, independent facilitator, community activist and Ambassador for Public Appointments.

David Gilbert is a former mental health service user, a Leeds United supporter and director of InHealth Associates, which supports organisations and individuals in turning patient and public engagement and co-production into everyday practice. Current initiatives include developing The Centre for Patient Leadership.

Lawrence Goldberg is consultant nephrologist and chief of specialised services in the Brighton and Sussex University Hospitals NHS Trust.

Malik Gul is director of the Community Empowerment Network in Wandsworth. Through a 30-year career in front-line community development he has sustained a belief in the power of people to make a difference. Learning and reflecting within the Masters in Public Administration programme at the University of Warwick has enabled him better to join the dots between public agency working and the communities they are seeking to serve.

Mike Hales is author of *Living thinkwork – where do labour processes come from?* (CSE Books, 1980). He and Bob Sang, while colleagues at the University of Brighton (Brighton Polytechnic) business school, worked in some surprising places as allies in the cause of self-management and dialogue across communities, in contexts of information technology systems development. He is a former user of mental health services.

Kate Hall joined Monitor in April 2010, working on board development. She is a Fellow of the Improvement Faculty for Patient Safety and Quality, and a Leadership Fellow with The Health Foundation.

Paul Hodgkin is chief executive of Patient Opinion, a not-for-profit social enterprise operating a website where patients, service users, carers and staff share their stories of care across the UK. He was a GP until 2011.

Valerie Iles is an independent academic consultant in health management, director of the Royal College of General Practitioners' leadership programme, honorary senior lecturer at the London School of Hygiene and Tropical Medicine, and fellow of the Centre for Leadership Studies at the University of Exeter.

Jane Keep has worked at local, strategic and national levels in and around the NHS for more than 30 years as a personal and organisational development and change facilitator and consultant. Themes include patient and public engagement, inclusive working cultures, health and well-being at work, productive working, and leading as peers.

Alistair Mant is an author and consultant who has worked in public sector organisations all over the world. He is chairman of the Performance 1 consultancy and of the Socio-technical Strategy Group. His latest book, *The bastard's a genius* (Allen & Unwin, 2010), is a case study in inventiveness and entrepreneurship.

Ed Nicol is a consultant cardiologist and general physician in the Royal Air Force, and works at Royal Brompton and Chelsea and Westminster NHS Foundation Trusts. He has an academic and practical interest in health leadership and advocates a holistic approach to service improvement, utilising skills and experiences of all who use or work within health services to improve outcomes for people using the NHS. Ed was a Health Foundation Leadership Fellow in 2007–09.

Fiona Reed is a coach, facilitator and trainer, and leads Fiona Reed Associates. A main theme of current NHS work is supporting people to develop the resilience needed in the current tumult. Another is how to influence across boundaries.

Jim Phillips works internationally as a consultant on health behaviour change, advising institutions, multinational companies and governments in the UK and abroad. He helped set up the Expert Patients' Programme in the UK and has advised and overseen the development of a range of self-management programmes.

Tim Sims works to strengthen NHS teams attempting new or challenging tasks that will deepen their impact on the health of their patients. For the Health Foundation, he and Fiona Reed designed and tested innovations in leadership-for-improvement with clinicians and managers, which they are now applying across the NHS and internationally.

David Sines is pro vice chancellor and executive dean and Professor of Community Health Care Nursing at Bucks New University. He is a fellow of the Royal College of Nursing and received a CBE for services to healthcare.

Rick Stern is chief executive of the NHS Alliance and a director of the Primary Care Foundation. At the time of writing, he was urgent care lead for the NHS Alliance, leading a network of urgent primary care providers including most of the out-of-hours providers across England. Previously, he was chief executive of Bexhill & Rother Primary Care Trust.

Tris Taylor composes music and occasionally does web, education and social justice projects (including: http://bobsangopenspace.org). "Bob helped me to understand and practice involvement, which has profoundly improved my life."

Lou Townson has been an independent consultant in the field of learning disabilities for 18 years. She is a member of Carlisle People First Research Team and of People First Independent Advocacy (Cumbria) and a visiting lecturer on the University of Manchester degree in learning disabilities studies.

Jan Walmsley is Visiting Professor of Leadership and Workforce Development at London South Bank University, Visiting Professor in the History of Learning Disability at The Open University, and former assistant director at The Health Foundation. She runs an independent research consultancy.

Jon Willis qualified as a nurse in 1996 having previously worked in the banking and insurance industry. He is currently Ward Manager of an acute care of the elderly ward at the Royal United Hospital in Bath. In 2009, he won a place on the Health Foundation Leadership scheme and for three months led the work stream on patient safety.

John Worth is founder of Know Your Own Health, an online self-management service. For 15 years he ran a successful digital communications agency producing large public behaviour-change campaigns and digital communications systems (websites etc) including many for the NHS.

Acknowledgements

A book in response to the sad and untimely loss of Bob Sang could not conceivably be made without contributions from many people in his wide and vital networks. In addition to the contributors whose chapters appear here – all specifically written for this collection – the editors also want to acknowledge and thank the following people who worked with us along the way: Andy Cowper, Graham English, Phil Greenham, Pip Hardy, Rachel Hawley, Sarah Pearson, Ed Rosen, Maria von Hildebrand, as well as contributors Valerie Iles and Tim Sims.

The book was initiated by Lisa Sang, Bob's partner, who convened the editorial team. We are glad to acknowledge the key contributions that she made, furnishing essential summaries and maps of his networks, commitments and ideas. We deeply appreciate the trust she placed in us as a team while we sorted ourselves out and got on with it, and the touchstone she has provided in occasional timely discussions over the past 20 months.

List of abbreviations

ADHD	attention deficit hyperactivity disorder
BMA	British Medical Association
BME	black and minority ethic
CCG	Clinical Commissioning Group
CCs	community champions
CDSMP	Chronic Disease Self-management Programme
CHC	Community Health Council
CIC	Community Interest Company
COPD	chronic obstructive pulmonary disease
CPI	classic professional identity
DEMOS	(the name of an independent think tank in UK politics)
EBCD	Experience-Based Co-Design
ECLN	Engaging Communities Learning Network
ELC	experience-led commissioning
EMIS	Egton Medical Information Systems Ltd
EPP	Expert Patients' Programme
EPR	electronic patient record
GMC	General Medical Council
HERG	Health Experience Research Group
HQIP	Healthcare Quality Improvement Partnership
IAPT	Improving Access to Psychological Therapies
ICT	information and communication technology
IHTP	Improving Head Teachers Programme
IT	information technology
LINks	Local Involvement Networks
LTCs	long-term conditions
MBCT	mindfulness-based cognitive therapy
MRSA	methicillin-resistant staphylococcus aureus
NaPaCT	National Primary Care Trust Development Programme
NEET	not in employment, education or training
NEF	New Economics Foundation
NESTA	National Endowment for Science Technology and the Arts
NIACE	National Institute of Adult Continuing Education
NICE	National Institute for Clinical Excellence (later National Institute for Health and Clinical Excellence)
PAERS	Patient Access to Electronic Record Systems
PALS	Patients' Advice and Liaison Service
PCT	Primary Care Trust
PPE	patient and public engagement
PPI	patient and public involvement
PROMS	patient reported outcome measures

QIPP	Quality, Productivity, Innovation and Prevention Programme
RSA	Royal Society of Arts
SML	self-managed learning
TDA	The Disability Alliance
UPIAS	Union of the physically impaired against segregation

Common abbreviations used but not in the list:
AIDS   BMW   CBE   DVD   GP   IBM   HIV   IBM   EU   RAF   NHS
PC   UK

Introduction

In today's hard times we need to think differently about how we do healthcare. Changing expectations, changing health needs and economic retrenchment together add up to an urgent argument for change, a call for the 'fully engaged scenario' that Sir Derek Wanless made so eloquently (Wanless, 2002, 2004). This change is now urgent. The sustainability of public healthcare and public service values is threatened by the belt-tightening of global recession, and compromised by a ferment of institutional change that is extraordinary, even in a culture that for years has been fraught with 'compulsory innovation' in organisational forms and funding arrangements.

But how to make these fundamental changes? Policymakers exhort engagement, involvement, co-design and co-production; but what do they look like in practice? The book seeks to ground these ideas through stories from day-to-day experience, where engagement and involvement are central, not 'add-ons' or extras. Most contributors write about what they know in practice, and have actually done. The practices they describe are not always entirely new. In some cases, they have been going on for decades, particularly since systematic challenges began to be made to the prevailing ethos of the welfare state in Britain: that the professional decides what is right for the citizen, and the citizen shows due gratitude. It is the different starting points and the collective impact of these practices that is important. There never has been a more important time to review and reinvigorate strands of thought and practice in the fields of co-production, full engagement and citizen activism. This book sets out to demonstrate what these well-worn clichés mean when fleshed out in practice, and it communicates the excitement and enthusiasm of those who do this.

The book weaves together the voices of three groups. There are people whose well-being substantially depends on public healthcare services (and those who advocate for and support them); there are people who provide healthcare and those who give them professional support in continuously improving their services; and there are people who 'do management' in healthcare institutions (with or without the word 'manager' in their job titles). Some of our contributors write regularly for publication. Most do not. They are activists and front-line service providers writing to engage and inform others and promote better practice.

The inspiration for the book

The book owes its genesis to a very special person, Bob Sang. His sudden and unexpected death in 2009 closed a 15-year career in leadership and organisational development in and around the NHS, and an active and innovative commitment to advocacy for patients and service users going back more than 30 years. At the time of his death, Bob occupied the UK's first (so far, the only) Chair of Patient and Public Involvement, at London South Bank University.

Bob believed in developing the capacity for self-management – and, through this, the well-being – of people whose lives are enmeshed with healthcare institutions. The readings in this book are designed to ensure that Bob's ideas and inspiration continue to inspire others. You do not need to have known him to get a great deal of value from the book – but in the end, you may wish you had!

Who should read this?

This book can be read by different people in different ways. Some will want simply to dip in, finding a topic that relates to their experience. There are some very short and memorable contributions: describing an experience, challenging thinking or adopting a particular point of view. Other pieces provide more detailed case studies or arguments. Some readers will want to take in a whole section at once, asking themselves what the message is, for them, in the context in which they find themselves. Other readers might want to bring together chapters from different sections – certainly, there are cross-cutting themes that can be explored. We think the book will work particularly well in opening windows on worlds of practice for students, giving them down-to-earth examples to put alongside the critiques of policy and practice that they will find in the more academic literature. As readers become familiar with the book, they will be able to use it in ways we editors had not imagined; we have provided an index to help in this.

Each section has a brief introductory page or two, helping readers choose what interests them. Each also has a concluding overview that puts the contributions in a wider context, drawing attention to some lessons that might be learned or placing first-hand accounts in the context of some of the research literature.

The book does not involve itself in a systematic way with contrasting theoretical ideas, or the career of concepts: active citizenship, well-being, innovation, co-production and so on. But it is informed by knowledge of these, and teachers will find material that brings issues to life in a way not available elsewhere. Although at times we have gone out to find contributions of a particular kind or in a particular area, the editors have not solicited contributions deliberately to cover public health, primary care, acute services, social care or other specific areas of practice; or to ensure that contributions come evenly from across the UK.

Largely, contributors are people with first-hand experience of working with Bob Sang. That is apparent at various points, as they write about how and why they did whatever it is that they are writing about. We explained, though, that it was not direct tributes that were wanted, but stories of better outcomes and better ways of working, which pay respect to his principles and commitments. Some of our contributors did not know him, and the work they are doing serves equally well as an instance of the values and practices that he aspired to.

Our readers are likely to be similar to our writers: activists; people whose well-being depends on healthcare services; and professionals, managers and workers motivated to do better work in difficult circumstances. We are keen to ensure that this book appears on reading lists for healthcare professionals and managers, either seeking to qualify or on programmes of continuing professional development. It offers all these readers a rich fount of ideas, perspectives, approaches and stimulating real-world questions.

The structure of this book

The book is divided into five sections, each with an orientation that was characteristic in Bob Sang's thinking and practice.

Section 1 asks: *What business are we really in?* It is widely acknowledged that the lion's share of time and money in public healthcare is devoted today to long-term conditions. Doing things differently, driving down costs and reducing complexity are vital. It is much less widely understood that getting the social relations between service users and service providers right has the potential to transform lives, services and costs. The focus here should not be on long-term conditions alone. Self-managing better health and well-being at all stages of life, and working together in local communities to achieve healthier lifestyles and life choices, are part and parcel of what is needed. The contributors know this – they give us examples of types of practice and ways of talking about long-term conditions that reflect this approach.

Quality is the theme of Section 2. Here, practitioners, patients and others each take ownership of what a quality service means for them. The redesign and the commissioning of services – in dialogue with patients and with their needs at the centre – is now occurring in a number of places, as the readings will show. Cost pressures make it challenging but all the more important to get things right. Learning from mistakes is also a key part of quality – requiring courage and maturity from all. Being able to account for quality in ways that are meaningful and accessible to different audiences is a skill still under development.

Section 3 discusses aspects of *governance*, focusing on what happens when everyday worlds and healthcare worlds confront each other. The gulf can seem unbridgeable and service users will sometimes decide to 'do it for themselves'; we have an example of people with learning difficulties successfully doing research and making it count. Advocates and intermediaries, however, can play valuable roles when everyone is outside their comfort zone. Small organisational adjustments and practical support for outsiders can pay dividends for service improvement, as several writers show. 'Involvement' and 'engagement' are not simple concepts to put into practice, but contributors suggest how to move forward, acknowledging the complexities that will be met.

Innovations in the exploitation and implementation of information technology (IT) are absolutely relevant to a vision of well-being and service, and contributors in Section 4 explore the question: *How can information technology work for well-being?* They take different approaches to harnessing the potentials of IT to enable participation and self-management, bottom-up development and service improvement, quality of care, and a managerial culture of caring.

Section 5 is about leadership among all this change, churning and 'compulsory innovation' in organisations and styles of working, relationships and expectations: pity the poor practitioner! Brought together with the focus of Section 1 (self-management in service-user communities), this gives point to the question that guides this final section: *What kind of leadership to support co-production?*

Finally, after almost 40 authors have explored these issues, a postscript situates their contributions in a wider context: of movements of thought and activism that address the state of healthcare and well-being in Britain, the provision of public services, and their sustainable future.

This book was edited by four long-term friends and admirers of Bob Sang, who came together for the first time with support and encouragement from his partner, Lisa. The project was made easier by the enthusiasm with which our invitation to contribute was received by many wonderful people. We are keenly aware of how constraints of size and time meant that we were unable to include all the drafts that we worked on with contributors. We hope that all who have been involved will value the diverse whole that has emerged, and see it as a fitting valediction for the man whose work it honours.

SECTION 1

What business are we really in? Managing and self-managing well-being

Introduction

Ask almost anyone in the UK about the system of healthcare. They will talk of the NHS but the image that comes to mind will probably be the hospital. Episodes of hospital healthcare have an immense and often life-changing significance. Of course they loom large. But the business of creating and maintaining better health and well-being goes much wider, as the contributions to this first section of the book show.

The section opens with three powerful illustrations of ways in which programmes (national and local, inside and outside the healthcare service framework) can transform both the lives of those who use the services they provide and the relations they have with service providers. **Nan Carle** brings together issues of labelling people (as 'service recipients') with the practicalities of budget control and monitoring, and illustrates the depth of the change that can occur as people are coached in new roles. **Jim Phillips** reflects on the nature and the effects of the Expert Patients' Programme – a government-led initiative mobilising the knowledge and experience of people with long-term conditions in order to empower their peers. The 'mainstreaming' of the programme has had intended and unintended consequences. There is a powerful message in these two contributions about the value of engagement for both service users and service providers. **Angela Flux** takes the same idea into a different context: health promotion. She describes a 20-year series of inspiring, imaginative and fun initiatives that have energised and mobilised groups in a geographical community to engage with their own health and well-being. She goes further, however, laying out factors that matter to making a success of them.

Changing the language that service providers employ is one factor that matters. **Jan Walmsley** takes a closer look. Her chapter explores how the words we use shape how we behave, and how deliberately changing those words can be a step to changing practice. It was activist commitment and vision, she points out, that brought 'the social model of disability' into the repertoire. Perhaps the language of this model might help to change the relationships between people with long-term conditions and services so that they are supported as people, not 'patients'.

Approaching the 'identity' dimension of activism from another direction, **Mike Hales** stops us short, wondering about the viability of the idea of being a fully engaged and active citizen in the health sphere. How will it fit with our inner balance for different ones of us? His account prompts reflection on the demands that citizen and service-user engagement makes, and the need to honour the rhythms of daily survival, and the rhythms through which individual people change and grow. The final contributor, **Laurie Bryant**, became an activist through personal experience of mental distress. He describes the transformation in his life when he discovered the power of partnership.

Editor **Ray Flux** closes with some reflections. He firmly addresses the title of this section: 'What business are we in?' Of course we want to enjoy the fruits of medical innovation and to get treatment when we are ill. But is the NHS a victim of its own success? Have we created a world of passive expectations – a pill for every ill – rather than one where people and their communities are engaged enough to lead in managing their own health and well-being? In all this, what is the role of our health service, and of professionals in and adjunct to the NHS? A basic assumption of this book, explored here, is that if public services reach out effectively to people with long-term conditions and enable them to self-manage, then the forms of co-working and the 'ways of seeing' one another that evolve have the potential to renew the tacit contract between publicly funded services, professions and people in the general population. What is currently happening in and around the NHS is a game with high stakes.

1

Money matters! Personal budgets and direct payments

Nan Carle

Alex uses a wheelchair and found he was not allowed to use his personal budget to update his wheelchair to an electric model, but he was able to create a support plan that included a job coach. Alex employed someone from the local Greek centre who understood his interests and cultural sensitivities. With his job coach, Alex created his own freelance training and consulting business. He learned to manage his business affairs and to grow his income. Alex had a good understanding of the personal budget and direct payment system and was able to drive his plan in a way that worked for him. Eventually, he did get an electric wheelchair but it took 18 months to save his money and find other sources of help. He would have been able to work much more efficiently and independently with the wheelchair he needed at the start! His knowledge and drive enabled him to become a taxpayer, and contributor to the wider community. There is no telling what he could have achieved with an earlier easing in regulations.

Gerald had a history of aggression and was not a popular participant at the day centre. With his personal budget and direct payments, he and his circle of support designed a seven-day support plan for a few hours each day. He hired a 'travel coach' to help him learn to travel on his own to local shops and leisure facilities. He now participates at local events that interest him, is part of the local economy and is no longer the angry man at the day centre!

Mary Elizabeth is a mother of two young children and had a short-term physical disability that meant she could not move around her house or lift more than 10lbs. It was expected that she would take two years to recover and would not work in this period. After considerable discussion, she was able to use her direct payments for childcare during the day so that she could finish her education. She healed much faster than the two-year prognosis and also finished her degree. She therefore did not need the direct payment for as long as anticipated and was able to move forward in her life with new qualifications for work, and with her family intact.

Each of us has a greater opportunity to pursue our own interests, express love of others, take risks and participate in community affairs when we are in charge of our own money. When others control our finances, it is their interests and concerns that prevail. The development of personal budgets and direct payments is at the very heart of self-directed services in social care.

Personal budgets include direct payments to the person and are managed by selected local authority personnel. Following an assessment of needs, direct payments enable an individual to use the allocated funds to develop a support plan to meet his or her needs. This plan may include selecting staff and using the funds to achieve what is important for one's own well-being. This approach is a far cry from being 'placed' in a service or being grouped with others considered to have a similar need. The examples that opened this chapter illustrate how people have used personal budgets and direct payments to pursue their interests and gain appropriate independence from paid support.

In each of these three examples, there is a sense of personal transformation. Individuals saw changes in relationships to family and friends, to their communities, and to the public system of care. Outcomes mattered most. But while the greatest strength of personal budgets and direct payments is their potential to be used in different ways to meet individual needs, this is also its greatest vulnerability. In our current economic circumstances, the use of public funds is under close scrutiny and issues of accountability and transparency are to the fore. Where it is hard to count 'outcomes', it may be difficult to sustain such individualised approaches to expenditure. As a consequence, it will always be important to record how money has been spent and to gather evidence that individuals managing their own budgets can be a more economic option than block contracts and group services.

The transition from the role of 'service recipient' to 'business person' is at the heart of this transformation, and requires a new personal relationship with money, including knowledge and understanding of income, the consequences of expenditure, and the recording of outcomes. This suggests that besides the financial transaction, there must be some sort of interim coaching that helps people imagine and find their 'best investment' of the available resources. This transition is particularly successful when individuals with personal budgets are coached to understand that managing their own money, procuring effective services and demonstrating accountability are a part of the new environment. The accountability aspect to coaching should also help the new business person to record or register what the outcomes – planned and unplanned – have been. For each person, there will need to be a change in expectations and behaviours to demonstrate the new world of personalised budgets.

In addition, both agency-provided services and individual plans funded from personal budgets may fail to realise the hoped-for gains. We have become accustomed to a risk of failure in agency-provided services, and we may need to be similarly willing to 'fail and learn' in individual plans funded from personal budgets. Encouraging citizens to plan and procure aspects of their own care must also involve preparing them to understand and share the risks in doing so.

Finally, it is important to reassert that it is often people's natural support networks that are key to their personal transformation regardless of how the payment systems emerge. This is because the role of government in people's lives is a matter of continuing debate in Western nations and while they continue to expect individuals, families and their communities to do more, they will generally have relatively broad-brush mechanisms for encouraging or requiring this. Personalising care to maximise individual potential and benefit will happen through drawing people and their networks into closer partnerships.

There remains a huge cultural shift to go beyond our 20th-century over-professionalisation of care. Personal packages of money and supported opportunities to risk and learn may move us across this chasm.

2

Mainstreaming a chronic disease self-management programme – reflections on the NHS Expert Patients' Programme

Jim Phillips

In July 1999, the government published the White Paper *Saving lives: our healthier nation* (Department of Health, 1999). In it, the government set out its new vision for improving health and putting citizens at the centre of care. The paper put forward the idea of the expert patient: someone who is empowered to manage their health condition in the wider context of their whole life. It cited examples of good practice by organisations such as Arthritis Care in using lay people to train and support people with a long-term illness to manage their condition and who seemed to benefit themselves from improved health and more effective use of services.

In 2001, the Department of Health published their detailed vision for a programme exploring this phenomenon at scale: *The expert patient: a new approach to chronic disease management for the 21st century*. This outlined some key underlying principles:

- The expertise of patients themselves is a largely untapped resource in the effective management of chronic disease.
- 'Expert patients' must become an integral part of the design and functioning of all local NHS services, not just of a few innovators.
- User-led self-management programmes are the principal route for creating a new generation of expert patients.
- It is the responsibility of the NHS to ensure that these programmes are in place, that they are developed and that they are sustained over the long term.
- New provision must be integrated with the work of other statutory providers such as education and social services.
- All programmes must be firmly rooted in good evidence governing their design and implementation.
- Feedback, evaluation and assessment of outcomes should be a routine part of the operation and development of the programme.

The programme chosen to be evaluated and provided to the NHS was the chronic disease self-management programme (CDSMP) developed by Kate Lorig at Stanford University. The CDSMP comprised six weekly sessions of around 2.5

hours and looked at how to manage the day-to-day impact of chronic disease on a person's life. The programme was already being used by voluntary organisations in the UK and was unique in its use of lay people to run the courses.

A key element of the course was integration into local support networks. It also acted as an empowerment vehicle: as participants improved their self-confidence and took responsibility for their health, they also began to question paternalistic relationships both with the healthcare team and sometimes the voluntary organisations themselves. For some professionals, this was very challenging and was seen as a threat to their role as the expert.

What effect did a national implementation have?

In 2002, around 100 trainers were taken on by the NHS and tasked with providing training and support to enable all Primary Care Trusts (PCTs) in England to run up to four Expert Patients' Programmes. This had an immediate effect on voluntary sector organisations, with many choosing to stop their provision altogether. In addition, with such a strong focus on a single model for the intervention, many other self-management programmes were neglected so that while the mass roll-out raised broad awareness, at the same time it may have hindered further development of other approaches.

However, by 2005, many PCTs had begun to integrate the programme into care pathways and the programme was also seen as an effective approach to broader public and patient participation in the NHS: people who had attended courses tended to have a realistic and clear view of how they wanted services to be provided. A common theme expressed was the desire to move into more of a partnership arrangement with care teams, with both sides recognising each other's expertise and working collaboratively to achieve the best outcomes.

Following the White Paper in 2006 (Department of Health, 2006), the programme was moved to a mainstreaming phase, with a new community interest company (CIC) being funded and set up by the Department of Health. This marked a turning point in the programme, with many PCTs abandoning their own in-house programme and commissioning from the nationally organised CIC. The effect was similar to that in 2002: programmes lost much of their local flavour and integration. Some also argued that externally commissioned courses represented poor value for money, as resources and expertise were external to the local community.

Those organisations that kept programmes integrated in the local community and linked to other community programmes appeared to offer higher social return on their investment. A study that compared the social return on investment of three Expert Patients' Programme courses (Kennedy and Phillips, 2010) found that the course most specifically targeted and integrated into local service provision showed the highest social return.

Has the Expert Patients' Programme been a success?

In terms of raising awareness of self-management and the concept of patients being empowered to take a partnership role in managing their health, the answer is probably 'yes'. Grounding that empowerment in a fairly simple and structured training programme – which is potentially self-sustaining because it identifies and coaches some of its own participants to become trainers – has also been an important development. However, looking over the history of the programme and the amount of public funding it has received, one wonders whether a greater impact could have been achieved if more time had been spent on stakeholder involvement and greater use of co-production methodology.

3

Health promotion – connecting people and place

Angela Flux

Health promotion appears at the forefront of many government proposals in health, particularly those focused on the young. Yet we seem more at risk of overeating, alcohol abuse, unprotected sex and depression than ever. While health promotion is the proper and serious long-term business of both central and local government, it is most often understood as campaigns of leaflets, slogans and posters, produced by professionals and authorities, to tell the public what to do (Eat, drink, sleep, exercise ... and engage?) in order to be healthy.

Health promotion needs to face two ways: towards the public to improve personal, family and community resilience to cope with whatever health and social challenges people may face, and also towards local agencies to shape settings and services with more health-enhancing features and fewer challenges. Ideally, a health promotion service brings these two together: agencies and communities co-designing and co-producing better places to live.

Health promotion is rarely seen in this facilitating role, yet without this engagement – where both conversation and action take place – health promotion campaigns and literature can simply create sound bites, litter and worrying background noise about risks to people's health. For those who are learning to self-manage their way through life with a long-term health condition, disability, frailty or social disadvantage, some sense that their local friends and family and the services of local authorities are partners on the same journey will greatly improve their receptiveness to health advice and progress.

The context

This writing is a personal reflection on 20 years spent developing a partnership approach to health promotion between the local authority, the NHS and voluntary sector partners in Hillingdon between 1990 and 2010. Hillingdon is the most westerly London Borough, with a long, north–south axis, transected by the Grand Union Canal, the M40, the M4 and other arterial roads to London, and it has Heathrow airport within its boundaries. It is at once suburban, commercial and industrial, green, and multicultural.

My journey began working on the prevention of HIV and AIDS in the borough and then, from 2000, on the formation of a joint health promotion team,

Healthy Hillingdon. In the 1990s, HIV was a high-profile public health issue nationally, which was being addressed across the health, education and social care economies. Its profile provided an opportunity for building fresh and somewhat unlikely links between the statutory agencies and community groups for the development of jointly owned prevention and care strategies. In Hillingdon, this involved schools, gay community groups, faith communities, drugs teams, local politicians and (often newly arrived via Heathrow) minority ethnic groups. Key learning points from this sustained programme of work became the foundation of the health promotion effort, which expected to:

- challenge and change the shapers of local society (bring to the surface and affecting the social determinants of health and well-being in the borough);
- mobilise and empower others to engage in this work; and
- work with members of the public individually and collectively to develop their own, their family's and their community's resilience.

Language matters

While trying to increase awareness of HIV and enable people in diverse communities to talk more freely about sexual health, the influence that language has in shaping our thinking became very evident. Shifting people's language and their use of negative, blaming words was a challenge. Besides the obvious abusive and offensive sexual terms, the language used by professions can also focus on problems and be a simplistic shorthand, when issues are often social, interpersonal and complex. 'Teenage pregnancy', 'obesity' and 'anti-bullying' are examples that have carried a national profile and are so pervasive as to have entered everyday speech. If we want people to engage positively in effective self-care, and to work with professionals on their journey to recovery and good health, does it help to use language that labels people as problems and their behaviour as targets for improvement?

We decided to use the name Healthy Hillingdon instead of 'the specialist health promotion service' because it simply named the goal and the place where we aimed to work with local people. Subsequently, the *Healthy* brand – as in Healthy Schools, Healthy Walks and so on – helped people to make the connection between programmes of work that they would not necessarily associate with health promotion of the leaflet and campaign type.

Throughout our work, we engaged with a broad range of statutory agencies to raise awareness of their impact on local health and well-being, and this diluted the tendency to use 'medical and disease' language in discussions about improving health. Indeed, a key signal that we were at the frontiers of where we wanted to be (and in the right place) was when people initially asked 'What are you doing here?' but subsequently came to understand something of the health and well-being impact of their planning work on green spaces, transport or libraries in the borough.

Engaging people matters

Securing cross-party political support, and connecting those affected or interested from diverse groups within the local communities, had been essential to effective education for HIV prevention. People with HIV were centrally involved in designing education programmes, which gave this public health issue a personal focus: people's experiences and their contributions as equal stakeholders mattered.

During this period, the Peer Education Programme was developed. It trained and supported young people to become central to schools' programmes promoting healthier decision-making about sexual behaviour among young people. Those working on the programme also valued and learned a great deal about what it was like to be young in Hillingdon and how to make their work effective. Learning from the Peer Education Programme was in turn foundational to the design of befriending and buddying work in schools and the cross-generational work that followed.

Networking across boundaries in this way to develop a health and education partnership proved invaluable in 2000 when there was a commitment to form Healthy Hillingdon, a joint health promotion service. People in the community continued to contribute to the education of professionals and other community groups, as the team developed the use of collaborative action learning, where groups in the community and departments within the statutory agencies worked together to envision and co-design programmes to improve local well-being.

In Hillingdon, it is not just settled people's experiences that matter: the borough has a constant influx of migrants, refugees and a history of travellers arising from its location and transport routes. Healthy Hillingdon aimed to value the contributions of all those we were working with, even when people had limited resources or very different perspectives. Particularly important has been listening to different people's perceptions of what health and wellness mean to them at different stages in their journey. This meant that inclusivity and valuing diversity had to 'come off the policy page' and characterise how the team interrelated with each other and with our wider partners and communities.

Sense of place matters

Drawing maps that show relative deprivation, pollution and need, by area, is widespread in the public services and has some value as analysis. Systematically seeking out and recognising the assets in a community is less common but can be a significant step towards seeing differently and co-creating solutions. Developing a positive sense of place emerged as a key part of our approach.

One of the earliest achievements in this respect was using Heathrow as a positive asset in the borough. In those days, the road entrance to Terminals One, Two and Three passed by a landmark, large-scale model of Concorde. A similarly large-scale HIV/AIDS red ribbon around the world famous droop snoot of this iconic plane made a considerable impact locally and internationally. This positive sense of place continues to help the people of Hillingdon to see their borough as a gateway to the world and a reason to celebrate our connectedness and rich diversity of cultures.

Since then, our Healthy Schools programme has enabled schools to build links with libraries, schools, allotments and parks, and has brought many different people to share working towards schools' accreditation and celebrating in their successes. A teddy bears' picnic event in our programme to reclaim parks for the local communities brought more than a thousand grandparents, parents and children from different communities and ethnic backgrounds together to share in the occasion. RAF Northolt opened its premises to local people to celebrate our Festival of Flight project, which aimed to build a sense of place (RAF Uxbridge is famous for coordinating the Battle of Britain 'few') and link children and families from very multicultural backgrounds.

Through these and many similar events, we learned to promote positive asset-based thinking about issues, which promotes 'can-do' action. Our approaches draw upon the concepts of pro-social norming and asset-based community development, while encouraging opportunities for valuing informal learning to develop community cohesion.

Vision and values matter

Like community development, progress in health promotion happens relatively slowly. The vision has to be sustained through political turbulence, restructuring, target-chasing and budgetary constraint. Although core funding is a mark of political commitment, a broad-based resource pool of funding, personnel and contacts helped sustain vision and momentum. Our aim was to pilot programmes successfully in local neighbourhoods where opportunities presented, and to profile them more widely to encourage similar initiatives elsewhere. Our Healthy Hillingdon branding helped people to make connections between diverse local events and to find the common values and aims from different settings. The variety of examples connected by brand name and approach encouraged people to imagine new ventures as opportunities arose. This variety of local actions made the programme more robust when individual departments or agencies went through inevitable periods of organisational turbulence.

Being positive, upbeat and aspirational can be challenging through these times, but our team was held together by common values and a common approach rather than professional discipline or organisational structure, and this helped to maintain cohesion and momentum. We were constantly challenged by the tendency of systems to drift towards the safe ground of focusing upon treatment, care and service provision (where activity can be counted) rather than prevention and investment in early intervention, which produces greater gain, but in the longer term.

Creativity and fun matter

Reporting to the Foresight project on mental capital and well-being, the New Economics Foundation recognised that:

> Feelings of happiness, contentment, enjoyment, curiosity and engagement are characteristic of someone who has a positive experience of their life…. Experiencing positive relationships, having control over one's life and having a sense of purpose are all important attributes of wellbeing. (Aked et al, 2008)

Part of maintaining the positive experience involved constantly seeking new partners to work with on co-designed ventures. Their freshness helped bring periodic successes to a long-term direction of travel.

In one period, we began ensuring that the libraries in the borough were seen as a community resource. Samba dancing, talks and walks, children's art exhibitions, and library recruitment outreaches to schools all helped to secure the libraries' future in the borough and reinforce their local ownership. Librarians' roles broadened and local people knew they could access a broad range of information and services. Mutual confidence, service relationships and health literacy all benefited, and these in turn boosted creativity and willingness to embrace risk and share resources in thinking about local well-being for the future.

To promote registration with dentists and awareness that child dental health was free among a very multicultural section of the population, we arranged for children in the neighbourhood to provide an aerial photograph of them as a smiley face; this was used as the logo for literature and local programmes. It featured on the local Trust calendar used across the borough.

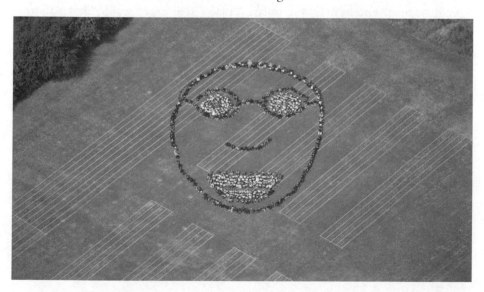

Bringing it together – Yeading Junior School

Many of the principles and practices of our work have been piloted and embedded at Yeading Junior School in the south of the borough. The area was often described by professionals as having high social needs. The school had relatively low levels of parental engagement, high levels of local unemployment, many cultures and first languages spoken in the local neighbourhood, and potential for conflict and social isolation. There were limited connections between the school and other organisations in the area.

For several years, the head teacher, working with Healthy Hillingdon, has actively included parents, staff, children, other local schools, agencies and community groups to build an exemplary school and a valuable hub of learning in the community. In a few intense years (which have seen the school remain in its bounded and relatively old grounds and buildings), the school has developed a substantial and well-supported social education programme. It has a community house where isolated parents can find friends, and professionals are happy to go to learn and offer support and advice. Both the school and the house are regularly cited as examples of best practice nationally by the Department for Education and Skills and more widely.

One of our team was seconded to support the community engagement, which has been diverse and varied. Examples include:

- well attended festivals and celebrations;
- partnering with Brunel and Bucks New Universities, which helps to raise children's and parents' aspirations;
- being the first school in the UK to pilot the Families and Schools Together programme;
- regular involvement in community events such as peace walks, interfaith peer education and the Festival of Flight; and
- having a Pyramid Club scheme in place throughout the school.

The school was the only primary school in the borough to be the hub and to lead a cluster of eight schools, which greatly enhanced the sharing of ideas and resources and the transition of children from primary to secondary education.

Parents have become more involved in the school, sensing that it is their place too. They embarked upon their own learning journeys, becoming both more independent and more engaged: able to organise and orchestrate events for the school and its associated community. As the community network has strengthened, this has contributed to better educational achievement among the children, which is currently clearly exceeding the national average.

In conclusion

Health promotion in Hillingdon has taken a journey. From the ground being prepared by working on one sensitive public health issue (HIV), it has engaged people at all levels and in many agencies across the borough. It has kept people and their perceptions of health and well-being to the fore, always seeking to adopt positive language and naming programmes by the positive goals being sought. The team of people involved has grown and been identified mainly by their common values, vision and approach, rather than by professional discipline or department. Where the work has been effective, boundaries of organisation and role have tended to be fuzzy. Health promotion has aimed to influence the shapers of local society where their impact on local people's health was not initially evident. We have been playing the long game but have aimed to make it fun and sustainable along the way!

4

Is a long-term condition a disability? Schools of thought and language

Jan Walmsley

One of the challenges we face in creating new ways of thinking about public services and healthcare systems is finding the right language. What do we call the people traditionally known as patients, service users or clients? All these terms convey a sense of passivity. None hints at mutuality, reciprocity or the dialogue advocated by many contributors.

It has been a problem, not because we want to dance on academic pin heads, but because language shapes the way we think and act. Finding language that encapsulates changed relationships between provider and recipient is a matter of urgency. In considering this challenge, my instinct was to look at the radicals of the disability movement, who have apparently changed the way we think about disability: from being an individual tragedy, to being something largely created by societal barriers. Are there similar lessons to be learnt and applied more widely, to 'people with long-term conditions' for example?

How 'long-term conditions' are framed

The discipline of medical sociology has dominated the way the impact of 'chronic illness' – what we now term 'long-term conditions' – has been studied. Influential ideas about the role of medicine as a way of controlling a common form of deviance in society – illness – were developed by Talcott Parsons, a sociologist publishing in the 1950s. Whereas healthy people (according to this view) fulfil their functions as paid and unpaid workers, sick people opt out of contributory roles. A healthy society requires illness to be managed in such a way that individuals are restored to health. Medicine's part is to legitimise the sick role temporarily, by signing sick notes and the like, on condition that sick people follow doctors' orders and return to normal functioning as soon as possible. Even individuals with chronic/long-term illnesses are expected to optimise functioning by following the prescribed regimen (Parsons, 1975).

Researchers into the way individuals respond to the onset of chronic illness have emphasised the need for them to manage and adapt, not just in practical ways, but also in the acquisition of a new, unwelcome and spoiled identity. Lifestyles have to be redesigned, homes adapted, jobs abandoned or renegotiated, even new wardrobes must sometimes be purchased:

> The sick person has to learn the pattern of his [sic] symptoms: when they appear, how long they last, whether he can prevent them, whether he can shorten their duration or minimise their intensity – and whether he is getting new ones. (Strauss and Glaser, 1975)

For medical sociologists, the onus is on the person: to juggle, relearn, adapt, negotiate and cope. Medicine legitimises their withdrawal from social roles and, in return, 'patients' are expected to conform to treatment, get better and get back to productive life as workers, parents and so on. These ideas remain embedded in the way we think about long-term conditions (LTCs) half a century on.

The new vision of care for people with LTCs, expressed in policy documents, is to:

> [Combine] much greater involvement of patients in their own care, with better co-ordinated and personalised care. People will be helped to take responsibility for their own health, including how to prevent, detect and treat their illnesses. There will be rapid diagnosis with early interventions, provided closer to home, with patients as lead partners in decisions. All interventions will be co-ordinated around the patient, and accessible at their convenience. (NHS West Midlands, 2008, p 1)

Thus, it is hoped, the person becomes less passive and more able to influence the way their care is delivered and the way they live their lives. Nevertheless, Talcott Parsons' sick role is embedded there. The patient is still a patient, expected to cooperate and to do their bit in getting back to full functionality by taking more responsibility for prevention, detection and treatment.

How disability is framed

Disability is framed differently. Radicals in the disability movement argue that it is not the individual but the world that has to change. They argue that disabled people are disadvantaged, marginalised and oppressed. Disablism has been added to sexism, racism, homophobia and ageism as a form of social oppression. This all started, according to Carol Thomas (2007), with activists in the 1960s and 1970s, people like Paul Hunt who spent his life in residential care homes and who wrote: 'Disabled people often meet prejudice, which expresses itself in discrimination and even oppression' (Hunt, 1966, p 152). Vic Finkelstein went on to distinguish *impairment* from *disability*, defining the former as 'lacking part or all of a limb, or having a defective limb, organ or mechanism of the body', and the latter as 'the disadvantage or restriction of activity caused by a contemporary social organization' (UPIAS and TDA, 1976, p 14).

From these origins, the social model of disability emerged. It asserts that disability results from social restrictions imposed by society, not from the impairment itself. The barriers to the participation of disabled people are firmly placed in society, not in the defective body. Disabled people are oppressed not by their functional limitations, but by the way society is organised as if everyone is young(ish), able-bodied and independent.

The social model has shaped policy and legislation in the UK, such as the Disability Discrimination Acts. It has also led many to reject 'care', professional interventions and the search for cures as part of the oppression and devaluing of disabled people (Morris, 1993; Swain and French, 2000).

So where does this take our discussion of language?

Language matters. Chronically ill and disabled persons can be seen as unfortunate victims or sufferers. Once the label is attached, according to another sociologist, Erving Goffman (1968), a person becomes discredited. Unless the person can hide their discrediting condition ('passing'), they are forever consigned to an inferior societal position. Freidson (1970), an academic associated with the study of the role of professions in society, argued that doctors have the power to assign a new identity – mental patient, 'cripple' and so on – to an individual. This then becomes their master identity, and there follows a process of induction into the new role of being 'blind', 'deaf' or 'schizophrenic'.

These arguments have led disabled activists to reject many institutions of power – in particular, 'medicine'. They advocate that we pay careful attention to language, insisting upon 'disabled people' for example, rather than 'persons with disabilities', to point to the idea of being disabled by society. Similarly, there has been a wholesale rejection of the concepts of 'victim' and 'suffering'.

The more recent policy interest in LTCs sits between the traditional medical consignment of impaired people to victimhood and stigma, and the strident citizenship claims of the disabled people's movement. Arguably, these two worlds come closer together in discussions about the nature of support people require to lead full lives regardless of their health status. The disability movement gave the world the idea of 'personal assistants' to replace 'carers', with the disabled person holding the budget, employing and controlling their own support workers (Morris, 1993), and this has become the model enshrined in English social care legislation (Department of Health, 2009). The concept has progressed more slowly in the health world but there are flirtations with it in pilots of personalised health budgets, where people with LTCs use the money allocated to their care to decide how it should be spent (Department of Health, 2012). What they have in common is a neo-liberal assumption that controlling the money equates to controlling one's own destiny.

Conclusion

I have drawn on two ways of thinking about people whose health is permanently impaired. Medicine can cast people with such conditions as victims, people who must cope, manage, adjust and obey professional advice to get better or at least minimise the burden they represent. On the other hand, the field of disability studies starts with the perspective that it is society that must change. Cure is no longer the goal; rather, it is to enable full citizenship for people, not patients, sufferers or victims.

These two worlds are slowly coming together, or at least there is some learning across the boundaries. In particular, this is noticeable in the idea that giving people with LTCs more control over the way their treatment is handled is the route forward. However, I would argue that the language we use for people with LTCs – patients – has not yet caught up with this thinking. This implies a sensitivity to the power relationships embedded in words. We should, where possible, use language that re-engineers patients into individuals with agency beyond their sick or disabled role. What might this language be: how about *people*?

5

Life as an active citizen – full engagement, hard work and well-being

Mike Hales

I find myself wondering about the 'full engagement' that we're promoting in this book, and how it's consistent with the value of well-being. I wonder if it's another kind of workload that people are now expected to shoulder, as politicians seek to shrink the state. I have often been aware of how horridly, overwhelmingly 'fully engaged', I am in certain aspects of life: in the sea of emotions and expectations that are part of working for a living. I have spent uncountable hours and calories struggling to sieve it down to manageable proportions. Does full engagement just mean working a double shift? Does it mean hardship or ease?

Engagement in work and livelihood arises in our kind of society through what Marx once referred to as 'the dull compulsion of economic relations' (Marx, 1867, ch 28). In contrast, being deeply engaged with our well-being is elective. It arises out of a choice we make. And it seems to me that having the capability and freedom to make a choice like this is itself part of well-being.

My experience says that – to my great surprise – the NHS can help to develop this capability. After decades of slowly deepening trouble, dealing with the demands of working for a living, I eventually became engaged with NHS mental health services as what we now call 'a service user': presenting with episodic depression and anxiety and embarking on a desultory engagement with low doses of anti-depressants. Quite recently – sadly too late for my marriage and career – I heard about Mindfulness Based Cognitive Therapy (MBCT), which is endorsed by NHS NICE guidelines as a 'maintenance treatment' for patients 'in remission from chronic depression'. That is not me; it is how the clinical psychology establishment tags me. But fair enough, as long as it gets me what I need (*sticks and stones* ... etc). My antennae twitched, I checked it out; and, yes, MBCT was the real thing: sensitive secular training in proper mindfulness practice, not (as I'd feared) some awful medicalised, cognitivist rip-off of a centuries-old practical wisdom. I was down to my GP in a shot, made sure I got a referral and went gladly and expectantly on the eight-week MBCT programme.

To find the NHS offering a form of treatment so deeply oriented to well-being brought a fresh breath after many months expecting a negligible NHS contribution to my capacity for living life well. Thanks to the ongoing 'sitting' practice initiated by that two-month MBCT episode, one of the things woven into my days now is an increasing awareness of and openness to what Buddhism calls *vedaná*: the experience, at this moment, of pleasantness or unpleasantness, well-being or not well-being, half-fullness or half-emptiness. On the back of this kind of awareness, real choices can be made, moment by moment, about the well-being of myself and others.

After the MBCT programme, I became engaged in my local Mental Health Trust as an ex-service user, wanting to do all I could to advocate and support the wider provision and uptake of MBCT as a wellness 'treatment' within the Trust, and participating in the Trust's research and development. So, yes, I find that I am an active citizen (when I was younger, we would simply have said 'an activist') substantially engaged in personal and public issues of health and well-being.

I am engaged also as an editor of this book, with its agenda of well-being and active citizenship. And, in this context, I find that a reservation arises with regard to different people's differing capacities for engagement, and the way in which all of us move in and out of various 'engagement spaces' in different phases of our lives or our daily routines.

On the one hand, for many people almost all the time, and perhaps all of us for some part of each day, engagement in the passionate tides of working, social and family life is a central component – perhaps *the* central component – of well-being. This clearly is true, for example, for very many people who work in the healthcare domain and in the field of campaigning about well-being: face-to-face engagement with other people and their needs and emotions is meat and drink. (Perhaps they do tend to binge a little?)

On the other hand, for other people (A minority? Who can say?) persistently over large segments of time — and perhaps for any of us for at least a segment of each day – the opposite is fundamental if we are to be comfortable and well: retreat, in the sense of solitary 'soul time' that is associated with prayer or meditation; or non-attachment, a skill and a commitment promoted by traditions of mindfulness. These two dimensions – engagement and retreat – sweep out between them a great, rich landscape of feeling and commitment, within which people occupy all kinds of positions. We move between positions in all kinds of regular or chaotic ways.

I feel that the agenda of well-being – campaigning for well-being – must not make prior assumptions that privilege any positions within this landscape. Especially, there can be no assumption that (elective) 'full engagement' in either well-being or campaigning for well-being has to look or feel anything like the pre-emptive and mundane engagement in 'work' that our social order brings us. Work may be joyful for one person and dully compelled for another, passionate on one day and desultory on the next, fulfilling in one phase of our life and debilitating in another. But being a workaholic for well-being – our own, or someone else's – seems no more a route to well-being than any other kind of workaholism.

I admire and generally am thankful for the energy and truly hard work that I observe among health workers, and those committed to activism for well-being. I am less sure that the values of quietness or withdrawal are easily accessible to people whose lives are lived in that particular 'engaged' mode; I truly couldn't say, it's a foreign land for my kind. Is the value of well–being that we're promoting in this book able to compassionately engage the whole spectrum, and the ways we each move through it: engagement and retreat, passion and quietude, community and solitude, approach and aversion, fighting and accepting? Let's hope so. I believe so.

OK, that's a wrap. Ouch, my eyes ache. Now … deadline looming: what email do I need to send to the book's other editors before the day ends? What do I need to read or write before the Trust MBCT governance meeting on Monday? Am I sure I can do 20 minutes' silent sitting practice today, before I'm too tired to sit well? And check in (better late than not at all) with vedaná*: what actually was the quality of work and attention through the hours of reflection and writing that I put into this draft today – Pleasant? Unpleasant? Half-full? Half-empty? How does this activist's sense of well-being stand? What does he need … right now? What do my friends, loved ones, colleagues and fellow conspirators need, to feel supported, respected, in balance? Right now, before this day ends?*

Is *that* active citizenship? Is it work? How hard is it?

6

Genuine partnership

Laurie Bryant

On my own with my challenges I found it very difficult to survive and often fell down. When my wife joined me, we stood some chance but we still fell down, we did not get the right support, we did not get the right information and we found it difficult. But the magic for us began to happen when those providing my care (wherever they came from, health or social care, or the voluntary sector) stood alongside us and we began to have debate, and we shared views and ideas, and developed a partnership. We talked, we listened, we swapped, we discussed; we came up with suggestions and we formed strong bonds that enabled me to stand on my own two feet more than I was ever able to before. But I didn't lose myself; I am still there within that partnership; my carer is still there within that partnership; there was a definite and defined role for her, and the people who supplied my care could also see what they were doing. And so we still maintained our own individuality within our partnership – to me the success of any healthcare service is partnerships. This process enabled all of us to explore and identify what skills, knowledge and understandings we all brought to the situation and how each of us could take a 'leadership' role from our perspectives in enabling me to journey along my 'road to recovery'. I had choice. My choice! I began to lead in my care. How uplifting an experience that was!

This was the beginning of me becoming a leader, not only within my own care pathways, but also to use this experience in being able to lead in developing strategic service development both regionally and nationally.

7

Overview: Looking for a new social contract around the NHS

Ray Flux

In this overview, I am going to expand on a dilemma for the NHS, propose a new deal between the public and its public services as a way forward, and draw on the contributions made in this section, teasing out some themes further examined elsewhere in the book.

The NHS – a victim of its own success

The NHS is in the vanguard of the public services in the UK. Apparently cherished by voters and championed by politicians, challenged by its own success over the years and made profoundly aware of instances of failure by the media, it is constantly required to contain its costs while expanding its reach.

All this takes place with little or no transparent public debate about the proper criteria for choosing priorities or indeed what the future understanding is between the NHS and the public. Policy often esteems local decision-making and personal choice but puts up no strong rebuttal when lobbyists or the media lambast the national service for offering a postcode lottery in the variety of services and quality of care available. So, more than 70 years after the setting up of the NHS, we might need to ask again: what business are we in?

We could address this by examining the health status of the population. We know ever more about needs in the population that could be met, made infinitely more complex than could have been imagined in the 1940s by our technical capacity in medicine, surgery and genetics, and our sensitivity to the needs of subsets within the increasingly diverse and expectant population. This, among other things, highlights the difficulty of choosing priorities while there is no common understanding of, or mandate for, the criteria and method to do so. Meanwhile, we obscure and frequently shuffle responsibilities and mechanisms for decision-making on a population-wide basis, which is what the NHS calls 'commissioning'. In 2012, as this draft is being completed, commissioning in England is going through radical reorganisation once again.

At the same time, decision-making on a personal care level has become more and more the realm of the clinical specialist. There are many instances where good front-line practitioners now engage the patient and their carers in discussion about their care pathway in the system. But this is often foreign ground to the unprepared patient; and when they are most ill, they are likely to take passively whatever offer of care is made at the time. Thus, at both population and personal levels, we often struggle to understand or engage in the processes we have for deciding how best to use our health service resources. The NHS is popularly cherished but – by this token – hardly owned or 'in partnership' with its public.

Some hard-hitting numbers

We do not have to go far into the examination of need to understand now that the NHS not only has to deliver its high-cost rescue service to the acutely ill, but also has to deal with a population who are not ill much of the time but have a long-term condition that they need to manage and live well with. Two sets of numbers help give a sense of scale, and begin to indicate the challenge.

First, it has been known for more than 25 years that while the NHS is the largest employer in Europe and one of the biggest organisations in the world, its 1 million-plus staff is dwarfed by the estimated 6 million members of the public who provide the equivalent of full-time care. If we ask 'How has this resource been educated, supported, valued and developed in the years since this disproportion was recognised?', the answer has to be: scantily.

Now, set alongside this, another number: 15–17 million people in the UK population live with a long-term condition – one in four: men, women and children, younger and older, isolated and integrated, wealthy and impoverished. With more elderly people and people living with long-term conditions, a highly politicised and scrutinised, audited and institutionally delivered, public-service-only response to maintaining health and well-being in the population will not work. We need to identify and mobilise more of the resources in the individuals, families and communities that sustain and promote health, recognising active citizens as valuable and valued partners. Again we must ask: how will this resource (these people) be educated, supported, valued and developed to manage their health (their lives) well?

For many of us citizens, our health is a given, not something that we work to enhance and preserve for ourselves, on top of the work we do to pay the bills and keep daily life on track. A 'given', that is, until it is diminished or considered to be at risk; but, at that point, public services – universally available, largely free at the point of delivery – can reinforce this skewed view of the value of health as a 'free good'. No effort required? Further, the priority that public services place on fixing our health problems tends to confirm to us that they are mainly concerned with taking responsibility in times of illness and frailty. Our language relabels us at these times as patients-of-doctors, and our condition as disease (rather than as, for example, people working to sustain our well-being through our own efforts and resources) – with negative consequences demonstrated and addressed throughout the book.

Put bluntly, not enough people look after health; and public services take care of illness. This is a bad deal, and it is unsustainable.

Mass movement – cogs in the healthcare machine

Is this tantamount to saying that the public must up its game and mobilise their resources to save an unsustainable system? This is not an attractive option. But the national scale of the shift required does call for serious mass movement – of ideas, of commitments and of expectations.

How could this happen? What range of influences can be brought to bear – for example, in the realms of government, of healthcare organisation, of front-line professional service provision and among the public – to enable the system to keep working safely and more effectively given the changing nature of the task(s).

Governments and the structure of healthcare provision have significant parts to play in this but are constantly replaced (through the electoral process) in the case of the former, and reshuffled and tweaked through government intervention in the latter. These two cogs in a complex machine turn on quite short timescales; and, like small cogs in large machines, they can exert disproportionate influence. We recognise their power but are not much concerned with them in this book.

Instead, the greater part of the approach we are exploring involves shifting and rebalancing public and staff experiences of each other: changing their expectations of each other's respective roles, responsibilities and resources, and as a consequence changing their behaviour too. These two 'wheels' in the system – public behaviour and staff behaviour – are much bigger and turn more slowly. Changes will take time and can only be secured openly through dialogue, by negotiating a new partnership between professional staff working in public services (at all levels, 'managers' included) and active citizens.

Activists in 'programme space' and attempts to achieve national scale

The writings that open this book illustrate the variety and scale of some approaches that help. Nan Carle, Jim Phillips and Angela Flux explore approaches on a wider canvas that encourage and enable local engagement and learning in communities where many may have given up on schooling years ago (or had schooling give up on them), and where many also find that life is calling for an adaptive and real response to the day-to-day challenges they experience.

All three are writing from 'programme space': where the resources of some part of the state (state welfare benefits, NHS budgets, local authority budgets) are available – for a period of time governed by electoral and managerial timescales – to support local or personal initiatives (in personal services, the management of long-term illness, everyday approaches to greater health and well-being). The approaches have features in common. They embrace diversity, not as a politically correct incantation, but because people and localities are actually at the practical centre of their work. They pay attention to the language they use, and listen to people. They allow and enable people to assess and take their own risks. They guide and tutor them in exercising new skills. They seek to share responsibility, resources and power in partnerships; and they seem naturally interested to collect and share stories of others' experience. They recognise and would like to offset some of the downside of 'mainstreamed' initiatives.

'Stories', in particular – and the voices that tell the stories – are themes that continue to resonate right through this book: in Section 2, as drivers of service quality; in Section 3 making connections across 'colliding worlds' of social experience; in Section 4, exploring issues of 'cheap voice' brought into the foreground by digital media; and in Section 5, exploring how paying skilful and respectful attention to voices can influence the development and the action of leaders.

Nan Carle describes local, successful interventions with stories of three people: Alex, Gerald and Mary Elizabeth. These arose during her work directing a programme in which people with disabilities are helped to negotiate spending a personal budget, to procure personal support of their choice. Although they are successes, the stories show how sometimes a programme's rules limit personal choice. In a context of financial stringency, the programme was always under scrutiny to demonstrate value for money, and it emerges that teaching budget-holders to help the system, by furnishing such information, is an important part of helping them gain the benefits that they themselves need. Collecting and sharing stories emerges as a powerful tool in this movement.

Jim Phillips offers reflection on a field where research and evidence-based, small-scale practice were encouraging self-management for people with long-term conditions. These examples of good practice were 'mainstreamed' into a national Expert Patients' Programme (EPP). The government-backed national roll-out of EPP was only partially successful, since – under pressures of financial stringency and economies of scale – local support and funding for alternatives and for a diversity of localised approaches tended to dry up. The challenge of moving good local work to 'mass scale' is a significant issue.

Personally, I explored this issue any number of times with Bob Sang (whose work we are honouring in this book) without resolving it. We were aware that specific examples of good practice may work anywhere but will not work everywhere; we knew also that national systems need universal or large-scale approaches, but that systematising good examples of local practice almost never works well across the broad canvas. There cannot be a template answer. In good local engagement, there seems to be a chemistry and a history of people, opportunity, motivation, connection and so on, which local champions are able to recognise and work with, to move things forward – 'here' and 'now'. Angela Flux writes more about this in this section; Malik Gul (in Section 5) and Beryl Furr (in Section 3) also touch directly on it; and Lawrence Goldberg (in Section 4) refers to it in the context of national initiatives for information technology (IT) in the NHS.

If we cannot readily systematise and exactly replicate good local practice, perhaps we can build a cascade. That is, through education, networks, sharing stories and coaching on a large scale, we can sensitise many more people to think, speak and behave differently; sharing, in turn, their own experiences. Each response will be slightly different – hybridising, cross-fertilising, adapting to local cultures and histories. Working in this way is much more energising and may prove to be more authentic in any particular setting.

Angela Flux writes from within a local authority setting about work in a London borough over 20 years. Her chapter reads as a catalogue of success (which it is) but is also designed to illustrate the 'can do' and 'how to' of this kind of journey. Phillips and Carle give accounts of their success tempered with some challenges. Flux sets out in a systematic and confident way the things that matter ('creativity and fun matter', 'language matters' and so on) in building an enduring dynamic, an engagement with communities and a constantly growing resource base. But this systematic catalogue hints at the opposition and difficulty the team faced and the learning they have accumulated over 20 years: people 'just not getting' the approach, continuous restructuring of local government and national organisations, budgetary constraints, and the tendency to do the safe or the urgent target-chasing thing.

Angela Flux's chapter illustrates in greatest detail what it takes to maintain a cultural shift over the long term. Champions often have to stay in one locality for a while and, even so, must build and rebuild a broad base of people with shared values and understanding of the approach if they are to withstand the turbulence of political and structural changes, target-chasing and budgetary squeeze. 'Having history in a place' may be needed before a local leader knows about opportunities, and who or what are the less obvious shapers of local culture. Such work, while often opportunistic, needs to be on a broad front and with the long term in mind.

The micro-scale – activist identity and activist practice

This section's first three contributors wrote from their own activism in support of citizen and service-user activism, in the 'programme space' of public service provisions. The remaining contributions come from a different direction, and provide the merest sketch of a very large and complex field of issues to do with the 'activist' identity and the sustainability of activism for individual citizens and service users.

Jan Walmsley searches in the activist tradition of 'disability' for potential resources that might be exploited in addressing the even more widespread situation of people with long-term conditions. She proposes that the terms used in medical thinking about physical impairment on the one hand, and social model thinking on the other, influence how we think about and treat people. Social models suggest that it is society's response that disables a person whose body (or mind) has an impairment; a proper response to disability, in this frame, is change in society. Medicine, in contrast, focuses on treating 'a disease' in a person, thus almost making the person irrelevant (merely a case of a disease). Walmsley is asking: can the activist tradition of the disabled people's movement help in reshaping identity for a person living with a long-term condition and seeking to achieve and sustain well-being? This resonates with the approach to health promotion described by

Flux, which sought both to empower individuals and groups and also to facilitate their engagement and influence with the planners and shapers of a broad range of local services and settings.

Mike Hales takes another tack. He found himself surprised and thankful that the NHS provided a service that really helped deal with long-standing emotional trouble; and has become involved in a limited way within the NHS as an activist, locally advocating for this kind of service and providing a service-user perspective in settings otherwise occupied solely by clinicians. He wonders whether traditions of activism might not be forms of the same 'workaholic' trouble that he has long been seeking to escape, and appeals to a compassionate sense of well-being that embraces actions and personal strategies across 'a great, rich landscape of feeling and commitment, within which people occupy all kinds of positions'. He certainly stands opposed to the passivism of the medical model, and the expectation that patients will be grateful for what it is that professionals find themselves in a position to offer, but he also requires respect for quietness and even for something amounting to retreat in a campaigning world that wants to insist on 'full engagement'.

Laurie Bryant furnishes another example of becoming an activist. Discovering the power of partnership put him in control of his 'care' and started him on a road to changing the world on a bigger canvas. His testimony speaks of the potential richness of the health partnership on the front line, between engaged citizens and public service providers. Hales and Bryant are not typical; and there could not be a 'typical' episode that moves a person to become a healthcare activist. But what they do is prompt us to consider the diversity within the deep emotional dimension that may lie behind the activist experiences and practices that other contributors write about.

Roots of a new deal?

This connects back with the first three authors who wrote as professionals in their fields. A variety of emotional motivators may lie behind the innovations in leadership, education, engagement and service-delivery practice that are described in this book: for example by Carle, Phillips and Flux in this section, but also Goldberg in renal care (Section 4), Dale in cancer care (Section 2) or Craft and Stern in safety and quality management (also Section 2). People go down the committed, innovative roads described in this book for many reasons, but are often powerfully motivated to connect with personal hardship and suffering.

It can work. Making it work is the business that the NHS really needs to be in. A shift on a large scale is needed to bring about this transformation in the NHS's future contribution to well-being. National policies, infrastructures and programmes are part of this, but cannot do the job. Flood the field with stories that get insiders and outsiders engaged, thinking and talking – read on!

SECTION 2

Questions of quality –
not just ticking boxes

Introduction

Responsibility for the quality of services in the NHS has long meant looking
upward, using predefined performance measures and feeding information into
a national regime. This was true in those very early days of the health service,
when hospitals had to report throughput with a single measure aggregating deaths
and discharges, and remains so today, with targets and seemingly ever-changing
outcome indicators. Political debates continue – is competition a more effective
spur to constant quality improvement? If not, then what?

The contributors to this section are a long way from national-level policy
debates. Their feet are firmly on the ground as they discuss what it takes to improve
quality. **Jan Walmsley** looks at the question 'What do patients want?' based on
her afternoon as a patient. She itches to redesign services given the waits and the
waste she experienced. Two examples of improvement projects then follow. For
both, the hopes and fears of the patients are at their heart. **Catherine Dale**, as
an NHS manager, gives a thoughtful and enthusiastic account of an experience-
based co-design project around day surgery for breast cancer. It was listening
to patients as equals that made such a difference. **Georgina Craig** then turns
attention to an example of commissioning, where patient stories effectively framed
decisions about the what, where, when and how of end-of-life care. **John Worth**
writes in a different way, focusing on the depth of the cultural shift if we are, in
his words, to turn 'care' into 'share'. Although he does not quite put it that way,
anyone providing high-quality health services has to have the imagination to
understand what it feels like to be on the receiving end of care.

Safe, effective and up-to-date diagnostic skills and interventional competences
are, of course, the bedrock of quality, as the next two contributors are very much
aware. Behind the moving and indeed shocking tale of the death of a child told
by **Tim Craft** is the chequered history of attempts to manage medical staff, to
work according to protocols and guidelines, and deliver what the NHS calls clinical
governance. His message is about the power of a single story in re-engaging hard-
working service providers and reminding them that policy documents can be
positive tools. **Rick Stern** also offers disturbing insights into the daily practice
in medicine. We all have to accept that mistakes and near misses will occur – the
important thing is that learning takes place. We have to commend the courage
and commitment that gets this learning into the public domain.

The picture broadens out with our final contributions. **Catherine Foot** reminds us of the importance of keeping track. She examines what happened when trusts were required to provide 'quality accounts' for a local readership outside the NHS. She uses early stage examples to think about just what would make sense and be of help to service users. A final overview by editor **Celia Davies** reflects on the implications of each of the contributions and the challenges to be faced as health services move into the next era.

8

A cataract journey

Jan Walmsley

The chief executive of my local acute hospital is a charming woman and has done a fairly good job of restoring its tarnished reputation. Recently, I had the opportunity to attend a prestigious event to hear her speak about the leadership challenges of delivering better quality at lower cost. As I listened, I fell to thinking about my recent experience at the hospital she runs.

I had been referred by my optician who had noticed the cataract. My GP was happy to refer me on for the operation without seeing me. She sent me the Choose and Book form and I chose my local hospital, which has a good reputation for eye surgery. Although the wait was much longer than for a slightly more distant private provider, the operation had gone well, and my sight was much improved. If I had had the opportunity to complete a Patient Reported Outcome Measures (PROMS) questionnaire, such as they offer for hip and knee replacements, varicose veins, and hernias, I would have been able to give a positive account. The trouble was, the process was protracted and unpleasant, and unnecessarily costly both to me and, I presume, to the hospital.

It was my post-operative visit. The appointment time came by letter. It was scheduled for a time when I was on holiday. I needed to find time to phone them, and then came another letter with a new time. Luckily, this was one I could make, but this had all taken a week, and the visit was therefore later than was seen as desirable.

To attend, I had to find a half-day in a busy schedule. On arrival, the receptionist pointed to a scrawled sign on the wall saying that they were running 45 minutes late. Why was this? They must hold this clinic at least every week and know how long it all takes. She shrugged.

Sixty minutes later I was summoned. "Aha," I thought, "at least it's all happening now." Not a bit of it. I spent two minutes with a nurse for 'vision' – this amounted to a simple eye test, reading the letters on the chart. There was no explanation or comment. I was sent back into the waiting area to wait for an unstated period of time – the coffee stall had closed before 4pm. I could not go elsewhere for a drink at this point in case I was called. Another 30 minutes went by; then I had two minutes with the consultant who took one look at my eye and gave me my discharge paper. Adding in the time taken to locate a parking space, this all took in total 2 hours 30 minutes. My eye is fine, the clinical outcome has been met, and I would not be happy if it had not been. But, if they had asked me, I could have suggested several ways that they could save money and run a service that I for one would have enjoyed far more, and which would have been a more convenient and more efficient use of time for us all.

Top tips for improving perceived quality of the service:

- Set up the post-operative visit at the same time as scheduling the operation – save secretarial time, postage and unnecessary delay.
- Give a precise time, based on experience of how long the process takes, rather than calling people in batches.
- Combine the 'vision' test with the nurse with the clinical check-up – train nurses to do this, refer to the consultant only if abnormalities are found or a cause for concern arises.

Or, better still, I could have been referred back to the high-street optician who had spotted the problem in the first place – that way, the post-operative visit could have been combined with getting a prescription for new spectacles.

9

Using Experience-Based Co-Design to make cancer services more patient-centred

Catherine Dale

I am writing about my experience as an NHS manager, of using Experience-Based Co-Design (EBCD) to improve the experience that patients have of cancer services in acute hospitals in London. In a nutshell, EBCD collects interviews and observations with patients, creates a short film, and shows this to staff and patients, who then decide collectively which of the issues to tackle. Small working groups of patients and staff form to design and implement improvements in the prioritised areas. I want to demonstrate how the co-design approach can make health services more patient-centred. Listening, reflecting, facilitating discussion and pinning down key actions are the key skills needed. They are the skills many people have already learned in facilitating change.

When I started on this project in 2008, I had worked as a manager in the voluntary sector and in acute NHS trusts in London for over a decade. Moving into service improvement roles in 2004, I had been thrilled by the tools and methods for getting a group of people together who are frustrated by the crazy bureaucracy of their working life, examining processes, cutting out waste, distributing tasks more evenly and making things run more smoothly.

These process-redesign approaches are hugely important; more so now when we have to consider how to reduce costs. But process improvement and improvement of the patient experience did not always go hand in hand. Working, for example, on the 18-week referral to treatment pathway, I found that an elderly woman was to be sent to an entirely different hospital, with which she had had no previous contact. It was a terrifying prospect for her. On balance, a couple more weeks of waiting would have been preferable.

Our co-design project in breast cancer services provides another example of the difference between process improvement and enhancing experience. When we asked patients to describe their experience for us and we listened for moments that clearly stood out as significant – either positively or negatively – one of the key elements that emerged was their experience in the day surgery department.

To give some background to this, the procedures and surgery associated with breast cancer have until recently involved an inpatient hospital stay. Improvements in recent years have meant that it is now the norm for most surgical procedures associated with breast surgery to be carried out as day-case procedures. This clearly has a benefit for patients as they do not have to stay overnight in hospital and endure the disruption. It also, of course, reduces the costs to the hospital of such a stay.

However, several of the patients we heard from mentioned day surgery as being a real low point in their experience. On the day of their procedure, they would meet with the surgeon to be marked up for surgery and to ensure that they were comfortable with consenting to the procedure. This took place in a changing cubicle with a curtain. The area had been designed for this purpose since day surgery units generally involve high-volume, low clinical complexity procedures and getting into a gown ready for their procedure speedily is the order of the day. Our patients felt extremely vulnerable and exposed in this situation. In discussion between patients, breast surgeons and nursing and management staff who run the day surgery unit, a solution was found. There was a nearby room that was rarely used in which patients now meet with the surgeon.

It is interesting to think about why this had not been addressed earlier. For patients about to have surgery for breast cancer, raising something like this may seem too trivial. Also, the only person they could tell was the surgeon talking to them about the procedure, who was about to get ready for theatre. It would not be wise to distract the surgeon. Even if patients were to raise this, the surgeons themselves may not have felt that they were in a position to alter the way in which space is used. Thus, it took a discussion with patients, surgeons and day surgery unit staff to resolve the issue.

I cannot overstate the power of the dialogue that ensues in situations like this to shift people's thinking about how services are provided. Discussion can generate understanding that is beneficial to all parties. The part that really surprised me was witnessing patients helping clinical staff to simplify processes, for example, arranging follow-up appointments following surgery. The surgeons realised that things that were frustrating them were also frustrating patients, and hearing that from the patients gave them the impetus to go back to their colleagues and improve the way things were done.

I think we overestimate our ability to think about the correct things without inviting patients to be part of a dialogue. We could walk through a planned process, for example, but we might miss something. The real way to do this is by discussion with patients. There is no need to fear the extra expense that patients' demands might incur. In my experience, these discussions often lead to a simplification of systems, cutting out the wasted effort of telling people about things at the wrong time for example.

It is challenging to measure the impact of this co-design approach in quantitative terms but I have seen people behave differently. I have felt a different atmosphere and I have heard a sense of relief in people's voices as they share their experiences and connect over what actions will be taken to address areas of weakness in services. I found co-design much more energising than surveys, where results too often sit on a shelf. In a co-design project, people see the films, attend events and discuss what has happened. Staff are moved to do something about the ways in which we are not meeting the needs of our patients.

I will confess that I had some doubts when I embarked on my journey of working with this co-design approach. I was cautious of the pain, anger and utter frustration that drive people to make complaints: the focus on one particular event or treatment period that seems to play over and over in a person's mind, not allowing them to move on. But EBCD is a method that takes patients and staff on a journey together. I went from being nervous about hearing the stories patients had to tell, to finding it an absolute privilege to work with them to turn their stories into priorities, to agree with staff which of those issues to focus on and then to work jointly with them all to turn these into action points that led to solutions. Patients can critique ideas before they are implemented so that we do not put precious resources and efforts into solutions that have not been tested out or at least thought through from the perspective of patients.

I recently attended an event in a mental health trust where a service user spoke about her experience of EBCD. She admitted that she went through a phase of thinking: "Here we go again, it might just be another one of those times that people ask for my opinion but don't do anything with it". The thing that pulled her through was the realisation that at the end she would sit down with staff. If that sit-down is well facilitated, and if those discussions lead to actions that make tangible improvements, what a valuable use of people's time and energy this can be.

Want to learn more about Experience-Based Co-Design?

- The EBCD model stems from work by Paul Bate and Glenn Robert:
  Bate, S.P. and Robert, G. (2007) *Bringing user experience to health care improvement – the concepts, methods and practices of experience-based design*, Oxford: Radcliffe Publishing.

- A useful brief chapter describing projects can be found in:
  Greenhalgh, T., Humphrey, C. and Woodard, F. (eds) (2010) *User involvement in health care*, New Jersey, NJ: Wiley-Blackwell.

- Catherine Dale developed a toolkit and step-by-step guide with the King's Fund in 2011. It includes videos from staff and patients from the integrated cancer care project at Kings Health Partners. See:
  www.kingsfund.org.uk/ebcd

- The NHS Institute for Innovation (www.institute.nhs.uk) also offers a guide and tools. See:
  www.institute.nhs.uk/quality_and_value/experienced_based_design/the_ebd_approach_%28experience_based_design%29.html

10

How patient stories can change the commissioning culture

Georgina Craig

My experience over 20 years in both the commercial and not-for-profit sectors in health left me feeling that the NHS loves to over-complicate commissioning. People who use NHS services are a huge resource and a treasure trove of insights into how to improve things – if only there were a simple way of tapping into this insight and using it to 'walk in their shoes'. On my way to collect my son from cubs one dreary October night in 2009, I heard Dr Ann McPherson on the radio, talking about www.healthtalkonline.org – a website for the public that shares people's stories and experiences of health conditions and uses a range of media, including video clips, to help people to understand that they are not alone in how they feel about their condition by providing insights into how others have coped in the same situation. I had found the treasure trove.

Since then, my social business and the University of Oxford's Health Experience Research Group (HERG) have been working together to develop experience-led commissioning (ELC). We launched the concept in October 2010 and published 'Introduction to ELC in end of life care' to stimulate debate. The paper can be found in the resource centre of the website www.experienceledcare.co.uk. A year later, we were nearing the end of our proof-of-concept work in end-of-life care, funded by the Department of Health, with Healthworks – a pathfinder clinical commissioning group in the Black Country – and an independent evaluation by the University of Westminster (Cheshire and Ridge, 2012).

ELC is based on the premise that good-quality clinical care alone is not good enough, and that by being led by the experiences of patients, we will deliver a great care experience at the same time as good clinical care – and that is what people say they want. HERG's archive of more than 2,000 interviews with people living with more than 60 conditions has been a key resource. As well as this, we have been advised and supported by Professor Glen Robert at Kings College, a member of the academic team who conceptualised the Experience-Based Co-Design improvement process in which patients, carers and front-line staff work together to redesign services (see Dale, this section). We have adapted this process for commissioning, and blended in ideas from improvement science – notably the Esther Project (www.lj.se/esther) – and concepts drawn from disciplines like cognitive and behavioural psychology, motivation research, linguistics, co-production, social marketing, and social movement theory.

ELC maintains the four basic steps of the commissioning cycle as set out by the Department of Health for England (www.ic.nhs.uk/commissioning). This helps orientate commissioners so that they feel at home. That is where the similarity ends. Instead of focusing on reducing costs, the ELC process focuses primarily on improving care experiences.

Commissioning is done over five workshops and undertaken by an ELC co-design team comprising local people and front-line professionals. Events are framed using 'trigger films' – montages of video clips of people talking about their experiences of care. Watching these takes participants out of their comfort zone and shifts the multidisciplinary commissioning team so that they are united in understanding and seeing care as patients do. It also legitimises the experiences of local people who tell us that watching the film is like "listening to myself talking".

Patient experience is fed in at every stage of this revised commissioning cycle:

1. **Needs assessment.** We contextualise epidemiological, demographic, cost and service usage data with our 'core' ELC experience insights and improvement themes, drawn from a specific secondary analysis of HERG data for commissioners. We run two workshops with local commissioners, patients and carers to benchmark and describe the local care experience and to articulate the great experience we want to commission. These workshops create a cohesive 'co-design team' comprising around 10 people – 50% lay people with relevant health experience and 50% clinical commissioners. They provide continuity and champion strategy development.

2. **Service specification.** In a workshop setting, a larger group develops a route map to a shared vision of great care in three years' time. Then, we work back to now and identify the first thing that needs to happen to get started. Any qualified providers are involved through an open-door policy. At a second event, we invite those who want to be part of delivering the vision to help create solutions to our improvement challenges and to pledge a formal contribution to delivering change.

3. **Contract design.** Once it is clear what needs to happen to improve quality, we invite all qualified providers to work with us to co-design the improvement contract and performance management framework that they will be measured against. This best procurement practice ensures that providers feel a sense of ownership and an equal stake in the final version.

4. **Monitoring and evaluation.** The co-design team meets again with providers annually to review progress at defined milestones along the route map. We also review feedback from users about how the care experience is improving. The cycle is complete at three years when we revisit what we said we would have achieved by then. We then refresh the needs assessment if necessary.

ELC is essentially about system leadership. It supports commissioners to open up and work with the assets in their local economy to create a shared vision and a new culture. By harnessing the power of stories, we deliberately use the commissioning process to engage people on an emotional level so that they reconnect with the reason they are proud to work for the NHS and for local people. Our experience is that the process energises, inspires and unites people. It is very powerful to watch. It is still early days. We want to trial ELC in chronic obstructive pulmonary disease (COPD) next, and across a number of CCGs. This will help us to work out how we might spread the approach.

Everyone's experience is unique. However, to be effective, commissioners need to be able to chunk up and identify universal aspects of care so that they can build a shared vision and improvement strategy. ELC is helping commissioners to do this. And maybe that is no great surprise. After all, it is the stories we share that bind us together and shape our culture every day. And that is exactly what we want ELC to do.

11

Turning 'care' into 'share'

John Worth

If citizens are to be properly enabled to make shared decisions about their care, language needs to be radically revised, the powerful design principles used in 'consumer' environments need to translate into 'care' environments; and the starting point for service redesign needs to be *what it feels like* for the citizen.

But how easily can any of us imagine what 'human need' actually looks and feels like? To be unwell, frightened, vulnerable, frail, disabled, abused, disenfranchised, addicted, to manage a mental illness or to be homeless? And how does it feel to be angry at citizen services that have as much ability to disempower us as they do to help us?

Whom do service organisations think they are serving? At some point in all of our lives, it will be 'us' and the hard fact is that the system as we know it now may not be there to support us in the way we would like it to in the future. Only by fully appreciating 'what it feels like' are any of us qualified to understand how we could re-enable people to lead enriched lives – whatever the life circumstances they are managing.

My central theme is that our understanding of what 'care' means and what constitutes 'citizen services' is in need of a radical redesign. To make an impact big enough to ensure that the public health and social services we need are there for 'us', now and in the future, we need to redefine the language and meaning of care.

Inventing more tools is not the challenge. The learning task for care service organisations is to figure out how the outputs from the tools we already have can be harnessed to good effect, to make them meaningful, relevant and useful, and to give them the levels of priority they need in order to scale them for maximum impact across wide populations. They need to invent the types of environment within which citizens can make sense of the services that are available, that help them to get the information and skills they need, and that give them the power to connect with others like them and people who can support them.

Careful use of language is important: service redesign activities that focus on notions of 'empowering people' and helping them make 'choices' are in danger of falling into rhetorical traps. People start off with power, the power that is imbued in their identity as citizens. It is only some other power that takes it away – like leaving them waiting in an Accident and Emergency Department for hours without meaningful information. Service redesign must start not with the ambition of empowering people, but with understanding how not to disempower them in the first place.

Furthermore, redesign starts with a commitment to authentically involving service users in the co-design and co-production of services. It involves compassion, recognising that people have personalised needs that are not helped by categorising or systematising them. Bob Sang made this point eloquently:

> A deep, taken-for-granted assumption in our culture is that if you have a 'problem' or 'need', you get a label: patient, user, client, sick, disabled, handicapped.... One consequence of such labelling is the separation of citizens into categories and groups defined by the service models that have been constructed to 'meet this need/problem'.... Very powerfully, at the point of diagnosis and analysis, individuals are defined only by their 'special needs' and/or their dysfunctioning, thus excluding their many purposes, roles, capabilities and aspirations as parents, partners, entrepreneurs, citizens. (Sang, 2007, p 45)

Design has the power to change our perception of what care means and support a paradigm shift: from services doing something 'to' someone, to becoming enabling services that provide guidance, advice and support as a pathway to choice (as opposed to presuming that choice is in itself enabling).

Design can create sharing environments – arrangements in which people are enabled to better communicate their needs and help themselves, thus contributing to their own care and easing the weight of care from being solely on service providers' shoulders. Design can also contribute to the workforce development needed to support such a paradigm shift: the way in which alternative approaches to service delivery can be imagined, visualised and potentially planned. If, within the education process, design is introduced well, staff themselves will begin to demand that the services they are delivering are designed better.

Fundamentally, if health and social care services are to involve citizens and enable authentic processes of informed choice, an overhaul of their culture of care is required. This will involve an overhaul of the interfaces they present to citizens; the types of intuitive interfaces people are now familiar with as consumers. And it will involve a cultural shift towards an unrelenting focus on customer care and great customer experiences – a big shift for statutory services where notions of 'my budget' and 'my target' reign, and where the language is often esoteric, focusing on inward objectives, rarely accessible to the citizens they are serving.

Care service organisations traditionally find it hard to take an unrestrained view of service redesign. The principles of entrepreneurship are hard to enact in conservative, often reactive, cultures, where the prevalent notion is that 'the system won't allow me to do that'. Care cultures can learn from consumer cultures. Examples of where design and 'what it feels like' are embedded in consumer cultures can be found in the way Apple designs its products and interfaces or in 'the John Lewis culture', where staff are literally stakeholders in the business, properly trained to look after their customers, and the goods are good, never knowingly undersold. How can similar principles contribute to the reinvention of the language and culture of care? The idea of great customer experiences is not one that will trivialise care services with corporate philosophies and the pursuit of profit. It is simply to point out that people expect their services to treat them well, to be personal, to know who they are, what they want and what they need, and to give it to them when they need it.

The Apple Corporation possesses what is probably the most significant example of a company with a ruthless focus on revolutionising the way we live. They use a pedantic focus on design detail in all their computer products to achieve it. We can thank Apple for the way in which we are able to make sense of information, watch movies, listen to music, share ideas, communicate with families and friends, and for tools that support creativity.

The parallel issues for care service organisations today are remarkably similar to those for the computer industry 30 years ago, when computers were largely mainframe systems. To gain access to care services today, citizens need to be plugged into a mainframe system, numbered and processed as part of the prevalent 'done to' culture. But the demands for healthy lifestyles and well-being are growing – they are embedded in policy – and by their nature they require citizens to be in control, manage their own data and possess the confidence and capability they have when they take responsibility for the choices they make on a shopping trip. Like pioneers of personal computing, the task ahead for leaders of care service organisations is to work out what the new interfaces will be and what applications will be needed to re-enable citizens to take control of their needs and improve their lives.

Leadership teams within care service organisations cannot afford to behave like command-line software engineers, addressing the future challenges of service redesign with an inward-facing focus – as though solution-finding revolves around single-dimension issues. To revolutionise their services, they need to participate in the move towards envisioning and designing something of the scale and significance of the 'graphical user interface' – an interface that will enable accessibility and personalisation for every citizen, whatever problem they are managing. Thirty years ago, when the demand for the PC was emerging, nobody really knew where it would take us. A few people, like Steve Jobs, were bold enough to imagine what the applications would be. Care service organisations will be forced to embrace innovation, make the space for imagining the future and become, not software engineers, but interface designers ready to give citizens the types of personalised applications they need and deserve. It will be the task of every leadership team to imagine beyond their current mainframe cultures. Increased prevalence of one or more long-term conditions, and ageing populations, mean that they have no choice. Failure to do so will leave their organisations unsustainable and unfit for purpose.

The starting point for tackling these emerging realities is to understand what it feels like, and recognise that every 'caring' transaction will need to be a 'sharing' transaction, characterised by better, warmer and more equitable relationships between citizens and caregivers.

12

Let me tell you a story

Tim Craft

Part of my job is to help lead the drive for continuous improvement in patient safety and the experience of being cared for at my hospital. This is important work but it risks being complicated and overwhelmed by the number of patient safety initiatives, guidance notes, alerts, recommendations and practice statements that seem to be growing at an almost exponential rate. One of the key roles of any leader is to translate and effectively communicate issues and priorities to the rest of his or her team. For me, that means communicating patient safety priorities with everyone who works at my hospital. My challenge is to make sense of this ever-expanding body of advice and ground practice change in ways that see a genuine improvement in the quality and safety of care offered to patients. Doctors in particular often seek evidence from controlled trials, numerically powered to produce statistically meaningful outcomes. The difficulty is that this can take years to complete. Feedback from patients or their carers in the shape of individual stories can provide a rich seam of opportunity to improve that can be mined much more quickly. Anecdote has its place and I frequently use patient stories to help everyone I work with see how what they do can affect safety.

Every clinician wants to provide the best and most up-to-date care for patients that they can. New procedures or therapies, however, need to be introduced carefully and safely. I often tell a story to help colleagues to understand the need for controls and governance around how we introduce new treatments into my hospital. It is the story of a little girl called Bethany and it is a true story. Beth was born at our hospital. Beth's mother knows that I tell the story and gave me a copy of a photograph of Beth. She too tells the story of what happened to Beth at national meetings held to improve the safety of healthcare.

Whenever I can, I tell the story using a slide. It is just one slide and it is the picture of Beth when she was about four years old.

Like other members of her family, Beth suffered from a condition called hereditary spherocytosis. In short, this meant that Beth's red blood cells were not the usual round doughnut shape but instead were shaped like spheres. The spleen of people with this condition works hard to remove these abnormally shaped cells from the bloodstream; it gets bigger and the patient becomes anaemic. Such patients are usually recommended to have their spleen removed and, indeed, many of Beth's relatives have had this done. Beth was referred to another hospital where specialist paediatric surgery was undertaken to have her spleen removed.

Beth's surgeons, I am sure with the best of intentions, decided to undertake the procedure using keyhole surgical techniques. In this way, Beth would have much smaller surgical incisions, a quicker recovery from surgery and a better cosmetic result. One of the technical difficulties to overcome, however, was that Beth's spleen was too big to be removed via one of the small portholes made for the surgical instruments. The surgeons decided to use a special instrument to, in essence, chop the spleen into more manageable pieces once it had been divided and disconnected from its blood vessels and so make its removal from the abdomen easier.

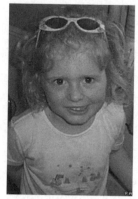

Beth, about four years old

The operation commenced and things were going well. Part way through, however, Beth suffered a catastrophic fall of her blood pressure that resulted in a cardiac arrest from which she could not be resuscitated. Beth died in the operating theatre, during what should have been planned and safe surgery.

During the ensuing coroner's investigation, it emerged that the decision to use the technique with the chopping instrument was made only shortly before the operation. Further, the operating surgeon, a trainee, had no experience of using the instrument (though other, non-paediatric, surgeons had) and it had apparently never been used previously in any type of surgery involving children. Members of the scrub team were not familiar with the instrument and Beth's parents had not had its use discussed with them.

A pathologist reporting on the post-mortem examination told the coroner's court that there were multiple lacerations to Beth's main abdominal blood vessel, possibly caused by the chopping instrument.

Beth's story is, of course, both shocking and tragic. It is not told simply for dramatic effect, though. It is told to support a bigger message or theme. It has helped my colleagues to understand the need to introduce new procedures in a safe way. Indeed, one of our surgeons recently told the story of bringing a new operation to our hospital using the policy as a guide at a large meeting. He stressed the assurance he felt from knowing that he was being supported by ensuring he addressed such things as theatre staff training and patient information needs.

Stories do not need to be as shocking as Beth's to help ground practice improvement but they are not just stories being told for the sake of it. They are real (ideally coming from experience at our own hospital), relevant to the change being sought and, whenever possible, told by patients themselves. It is not just performance scorecards or reams of statistical data that are a source of information. Feedback from patients about their experience and the content of letters of thanks as well as complaint are just as valuable.

A visitor told us that seeing the same spilt coffee stain (it was coffee, wasn't it?) in one of our corridors at the end as well as at the beginning of the day led her to believe that we do not run a clean hospital. Her perception was that her husband was thus more likely to catch MRSA or some other infection because a hospital that has dirty corridors means a hospital with infections. It does not matter that there may be no evidence for this. In the eyes of the perceiver, perception is reality. This is a simple message, but it is at its most powerful when staff hear it first-hand from a visitor. It only takes minutes, but we try to create a psychologically safe environment, where patients and carers do not fear retribution in providing feedback and where groups of staff can really understand how these small things matter.

We have recently filmed four patients who agreed to come back to the hospital to tell their stories of being cared for by us. These are not filmed interviews comprising questions and answers. The films are largely uninterrupted recountings of experience. Aspects of these filmed stories are then played back to staff groups and used as a point of reference, especially when we are focusing on improving patient safety. If anyone is struggling to identify with the message of the story, we ask him or her to imagine that we are treating a member of his or her family. 'How would you wish us to treat a member of your family?' eventually translates into 'What should I do to treat this person as though they are a member of my family?'. Often, these questions do not need to be asked; they are implicit when we consider the content of patient stories.

The point, though, is that relating improvement initiatives to real, yet relevant, patient stories helps us all to identify with the aim. Most importantly, it helps us all to realise that patient safety is everyone's responsibility.

Want to know more of Beth's story?

- You can watch Beth's story, as told by her mother, on video and see feedback from other viewers by visiting the website: www.patientstories.org.uk
- Patient Stories is a social enterprise that uses drama documentary film-making to promote debate about quality and safety among healthcare professionals.
- This 15-minute film was commended by the Medical Journalists' Association at its Winter Awards competition in January 2012.

13

Quality, leadership and moral responsibility

Rick Stern

People who use out-of-hours services tend to speak well of them. They are services coping with a high degree of risk: seeing patients often without any access to notes when in many cases they need urgent support and most services have closed down for the day. More than 7 million people are seen a year and while most have their needs met fairly rapidly, a few cases end in tragedy.

Two particular tragedies stick in the mind. First, the death of Penny Campbell in Camden in 2005, when eight different doctors saw the patient but failed to join up what they had been told. And second, the death of David Gray in 2008, when a tired German doctor who spoke little English on his first shift in Cambridgeshire 'unlawfully killed' his patient with a massive overdose of a controlled drug. Both these cases led to long and complex enquiries and led to pages of guidance for services across the country. While the recommendations are all valid in themselves, there is a risk that they miss the bigger picture. At the heart of many failures is a culture that stops putting the patient first.

So, if we take the case of Daniel Ubani, the German doctor who made a catastrophic prescribing error, it appeared at first sight that this was all about an individual who repeatedly failed to care for his patients. He turned up in a foreign country, unprepared and ill-equipped to provide safe and consistent care and the battle still continues to hold him to account for his multiple personal failings through the German health and judicial systems. What the reports and enquiries highlighted was that although this was about one individual, it also brought to light a series of system failures, from a provider with the deeply ironic name of 'Take Care Now' that failed to check or support a new doctor, to Primary Care Trusts (PCTs) that were unable to operate a system that was meant to identify unsuitable doctors. What was much less apparent were the personal failures of leaders within the out-of-hours provider to take responsibility for keeping people safe.

An 18-month inquiry by the Care Quality Commission found that this was not the first time this particular drug error had occurred. Twice before in just a few months other doctors had overprescribed the same drug, diamorphine, although the results were less serious in those cases. A doctor was noted as having told the leaders of the organisation that unless this problem was addressed, "someone will die". If an experienced doctor uses a phrase as stark as that, you would expect the hairs to rise on the back of people's necks and for action to be taken immediately. But the advice was ignored and nothing was done. The organisation lost an opportunity, and David Gray lost his life.

There is no reason to believe that those in charge of 'Take Care Now' were bad people, but they had failed to take responsibility even when they had been clearly warned that something was wrong. All the new rules and guidance may fail to put sufficient emphasis on this aspect of good governance: the fundamental responsibility to create a culture and ethos that puts the safety of patients first and seeks out and investigates problems as a vital source of information for improving care. In hindsight, their collective decision, or, more properly, their 'act of omission' as they failed to take action, looks extraordinary. But in practice, what looks clear-cut is often more blurred. The pressures of running a multi-million-pound healthcare organisation are considerable and, in the end, the corporate responsibility to protect the organisation may undermine a clear sense of what is right or wrong.

Let me take an example that did not make the headlines. As Urgent Care Lead for the NHS Alliance, I speak to many people who work in senior roles in GP out-of-hours services. A while ago, a former director of a well-respected out-of-hours provider described his experience in a senior team. He was on call one night and received a call from a call handler who warned him that she was concerned about a case in which a man had died after a request for a home visit; she thought this had the potential to become a major serious untoward incident. Next morning he listened to the tapes and could hear a very anxious woman saying that her son, a young man in his twenties, was having difficulty breathing and was very agitated, having recently been discharged from hospital after a major operation, and that she was extremely worried about his condition. In the recording, the young man's struggle for breath could be clearly heard. You could be in no doubt as to how the situation appeared. The mother said she really wanted the doctor to visit; the GP's response was "What good will that do?". He did not think it necessary to make the visit as the patient had already been seen earlier that day. He then went on to say that she could bring him in if she wanted, but by then the mother had taken his words on board and was reassured. It should be pointed out that the hospital team had not responded to her calls either.

A few hours later, the man was reported dead at hospital after being taken in by ambulance. The director raised the case at the next executive team meeting. The agenda was full, as always, of items about finance and business development, but he insisted that he needed time to share this case. It was apparent that other members of the team, some of whom had also listened to the recording, were not overly interested, with their body language suggesting that this was not a priority, or so out of the ordinary that it needed more consideration. When prompted, one of the directors said of the duty GP, "It's OK, he covered his tracks", as he had also heard the throwaway line: "Bring him in if you want to." There was little further discussion and the case was not reported as a serious untoward incident. It is difficult to contemplate the scale of public investigation that would have ensued if it had been, and the fallout could have been huge.

There are a number of points arising from this brief description of a potentially avoidable death. First, things do go wrong in all services, but when they do, there should be a determined effort to understand what has happened and review the case in detail. Second, leaders in health services should be spending more time looking at clinical issues, learning from particular incidents and looking at how to improve care so that any mistakes are not repeated. Third, although all organisations spend time presenting themselves positively and defending their reputation, glossing over or covering up mistakes is not acceptable. This case remained hidden. It is no coincidence that in both cases referred to earlier, key people close to the person who died had experience of challenging the system – Penny Campbell's partner was a journalist and David Gray's son is a GP.

The point of the story is that I doubt it is exceptional. I have seen in other organisations how quickly executives can slide from the public or patient interest to protecting the interests of the organisation they represent. Senior managers have learned that a central part of their job is to manage risk, and risk registers tend to focus on risks to their organisation, including their reputation. While it is essential that executives think about protecting the organisation they lead, it is dangerous when this becomes more important than protecting the people they serve. If we forget that each individual matters equally – that it could be our parent, our child – we cease to serve the public and, in turn, fail our public service organisations.

Most leaders in organisations spend too much time talking about money and business opportunities, and too little time talking about patient experience and safety. It is not difficult to see why. The rhetoric within the NHS may be about quality and safety, but the relentless pressure – day in, day out – is on finance. Leaders would do well to remember that few are sacked for financial failings – more are sacked when patient safety is compromised. There is a strong case to be made on a basis of selfish altruism, let alone an appeal to some wider morality, that we should focus more on what happens to individuals who come into contact with our services, especially those whom we fail.

So how do we help people focus on the things that really matter? How do we focus on culture, not policy or finance?

The NHS Alliance, which includes the membership of most out-of-hours providers across England within its urgent care network, established a pilot across 10 providers in November 2010 to develop a new anonymised system for rapid sharing and learning. Providers are reporting any incident where something has gone wrong and others could learn from what happened to improve patient safety and care, building on similar well-established initiatives in the aviation and maritime sectors. The format is simple, asking: 'What happened?', 'What did you do to address it?' and 'What did you learn?'. Reports of no more than one page, without names or identifying features, are submitted on a website and can be accessed by all staff across the 12 organisations. It is intended to work alongside existing systems for reporting serious incidents, not as an alternative to them.

Over the first nine months, 60 reports were logged on to a specially designed website, highlighting a wide range of incidents, all offering learning to other organisations. Leaders from across the providers meet regularly to review progress and test out and improve this approach for sharing reports on 'avoidable serious events'. It is already proving to be a powerful tool for individual and organisational learning, developing a culture where, as one medical director described it, "[There is] cultural permission to admit that occasionally we mess up". Another clinical lead observed: "It is the new culture of sharing and acknowledgement of error that is crucial … if sustained and developed it will evolve into something deeper and more important than we ever envisaged at the outset."

A major development for capturing and sharing learning has been the development of a 'clinical panel', chaired by one of the clinical directors with clinical leads from across the pilot sites. This is set up as a 90–minute conference call to reduce the time commitment for people based across the country, and focuses on a key theme coming out of the reports. The clinical panel looks in detail at relevant cases and tries to identify key lessons that can be shared more widely across the sector as a whole.

Hopefully, by shifting the focus to practical support for making improvements and protecting patient safety, we can have more impact than 'naming and shaming' or simply expressing outrage when things do, inevitably, go wrong. There is now a commitment to roll out this initiative across the out–of–hours sector, as well as potential for developing an initiative of this kind across groups of general practices. This is just one small example of how we might chip away at the prevailing culture in health services that leads to people at all levels 'covering their tracks' rather than shining a spotlight on our failures so that we can learn to do better rather than judge and blame. The greatest strength of the NHS is its people, who strive to do the best they can for the people they serve. Our systems need to be designed to support them to do this, maximising their potential, rather than acting as a barrier to openness and transparency.

Want to know more?

See the NHS Alliance website for a press release on a report: *Rapid learning: Driving up patients' safety across out-of-hours services*. Available at: www.nhsalliance.org/press-releases/article/date/2011/11/rapid-learning-driving-up-patients-safety-across-out-of-hours-services/

14

Accounting for quality – eight tips for producing reports for the public about the quality of care

Catherine Foot

> We will make the performance of the NHS totally transparent by publishing information about the kind of results that healthcare providers are achieving, so there is no hiding place for failure. (Conservative Party, 2010, p 45)

Governments around the world are putting more and more information about the performance of public services in the public domain. The theory goes that greater transparency is not only a right and proper thing to provide for taxpayers, but also that it will stimulate public services to improve. There is some evidence that this is true for healthcare (Fung et al, 2008).

This agenda is increasingly reaching the NHS, from many different directions. Perhaps the most well-known professionally led initiative is the cardiac surgeons' work to publish surgeon-by-surgeon post-operative mortality rates (HQIP, 2011). More recently, NHS London has begun to publish data on the quality of GP services across the capital (NHS London, 2011). Patients and the public themselves are also involved, such as Hackney Local Involvement Network's work to gather and publish patient and public feedback about local health and social care services (Hackney LINk, 2011). In terms of government policy, since 2009, NHS organisations have been required to write annual public reports on the quality of their services (called quality accounts) and, in 2011, the Chancellor of the Exchequer announced new investment in greater transparency of performance data across all public services (Cabinet Office, 2011).

But producing effective information about quality for the public is very hard to do well. There are difficult trade-offs and judgements to be made. How can you fairly represent quality across all your services yet select only a few indicators? How can you provide the explanation and context you need to give and yet be short and readable?

Eight tips

These tips are for NHS staff preparing their own reports on quality who want to produce something that the public will read, understand and value. They are based on King's Fund research (see the box at the end of this chapter).

1. Consult and involve your readers

Many of the first quality accounts produced seemed to be targeted at a range of different audiences, including clinicians and commissioners as well as the public, leaving them probably meeting the needs of all audiences only partially and none entirely satisfactorily. A document for the public needs to be written solely with them in mind. The same data can be used for internal clinical governance or board reports and so on, but that will require different language and less explanation.

Consulting with patients and the public takes time and needs to be planned in to the process from the very beginning. All too often, organisations can attempt some very brief and last-minute consultation exercise that achieves nothing. As one member of the King's Fund's focus groups put it: "What doesn't make practical sense is, if it's going to be published on the 1st of April, say, and you get it on the 25th of March … because … you've got no chance of altering anything in it, and it's just a matter of rubber stamping".

2. Try to give a balanced range of indicators

The 2010 quality accounts ranged from presenting only a handful of measures up to well over a hundred. The most common were waiting times, hospital–acquired infection rates and patient experience survey results. If you are trying to represent the breadth of services provided across a whole hospital trust, judicious selection of a range of types of measures of quality is crucial to provide an overview, however inevitably partial it will be. No one aspect of quality (such as clinical effectiveness, patient safety and patient and staff experience) provides the whole picture. Information on productivity or value for money, and on how quality varies for different groups (such as different ethnic groups), is also valuable. Different topics could be selected for particular focus in successive reports.

3. Be honest – include both your successes and your failures

While this can be difficult for some staff, and not least also for boards, to accept, a public report that suggests only the highest achievements and admits no challenges is unlikely to be a fair account, and will seem dishonest to the canny and sceptical reader. Patient complaints, reviews, investigations that have been conducted and improvement priorities that have been set by your organisation provide obvious sources of information on the challenges, the failures and what has been done about them.

4. Do not reinvent the wheel

The NHS is awash with data and information, particularly in the hospital sector. Wherever possible, reporting information that is collected anyway, for example, for payment purposes or internal performance reporting, saves time and money. It also tends to mean that the information is collected in a similar way, which enables comparison between organisations. By no means all information that is important to the public is available in this way, but beginning with data collected for other purposes is an efficient place to start.

5. Benchmark

A score of 75% saying 'yes' in answer to the national inpatient survey question 'When you had important questions to ask a doctor, did you get answers that you could understand?' suggests room for improvement, but ultimately is pretty meaningless without some comparison. Is 75% better or worse than average? (The answer is at the end of this paragraph if you do not know.) Is it better or worse than any agreed standard? Is your organisation getting better or worse over time? How does it compare with the service down the road? All of these would be valid benchmarks to provide some way of understanding how good your performance really is. (A 75% score on that survey question is worse than average, and indeed falls in the bottom 20% of performance nationally. The median score for this question in 2010 was 81%.)

6. Explain

A table of statistics is not enough. At the very least, your reports need to explain:

- why you have chosen the indicators you have;
- what each indicator tells you about;
- how good or bad this means your performance is; and
- what you are doing about it.

The language used is equally important. One focus group participant, struggling with a particularly bad example of a jargon–laden quality report, was forced to say: "I'm reading things here and thinking: 'What does that mean,"in quarter and accumulative trajectories"?' I know what they mean roughly, but I wouldn't … you know, who's going to look at it?" As another put it: "My advice would be 'KISS': Keep It Simple Stupid".

7. Present graphically but do so clearly and with narrative explanation

Presenting information visually alongside words can be very effective, but only if it is done simply and accurately. Some of the 2010 quality accounts had simple, clearly labelled bar charts, line graphs and diagrams, accompanied by short and simple explanations. Others, however, were a confusing mess of poorly labelled and overly complicated statistical presentations.

8. Make it easy to find your report

Many of the 2010 quality accounts were surprisingly difficult to find. Typically, they are available via the service provider's website, but are often hidden many clicks away from the homepage. If you are serious about your report being written for the public, then you also need to be serious about promoting its existence and making it easy to access, both online and through posters and other routes.

Conclusion

The Conservative Party manifesto quoted at the start of this section warned ominously of greater publication of information meaning that there would be 'no hiding place for failure'. But the NHS needs to embrace this agenda rather than be afraid of it. Greater transparency can prompt a positive chain reaction that leads to improved quality. Those trusts that have begun producing quality accounts report that the process has helped them to make time to review and discuss data about the quality of care and how they compare with others. It has helped them to agree priorities for quality improvement, and helped their Boards focus on quality alongside governance and financial performance (Department of Health, 2010b). In addition, opening up this process to discussions with local patients and the public can provide an even greater spur for improvement.

We are still in the early stages of a long-term, international trend towards wider publication of information about the quality of health services. But early initiatives show that this trend has real promise to help NHS staff improve quality.

Want to know more about the research?

The following reports are all available from: www.kingsfund.org.uk/publications

- *Accounting for quality to the local community – findings from focus group research* (Foot and Ross, 2010): a series of focus groups with representatives of patients and the public.
- *How do quality accounts measure up? Findings from the first year* (Foot et al, 2011): a review of 64 NHS and independent sector quality accounts that were published in 2010.
- *Choosing a high-quality hospital – the role of nudges, scorecard design and information* (Boyce et al, 2010): research with patients about how information can be presented to help people make choices about their own healthcare.

15

Overview: Quality – fantastic journey but bumpy ride?

Celia Davies

> Over the past decade the NHS has been on a fantastic reform
> journey.... There have been three phases so far, starting with a big
> increase in investment and capacity which has grown the NHS by
> a third. The second stage was the introduction of reform levers to
> expand choice and contestability. And now the third phase is bringing
> all that together to improve quality for patients. (Sir David Nicholson,
> in Department of Health, 2010c, Foreword)

Almost everyone who delivers care in the NHS and almost everyone who
plays a support role on the front line of care goes to work with the intention of
delivering high-quality care. And, for most of the time, they do provide good
care. Nearly eight in 10 patients reported care that was excellent or very good
in a national survey of acute and specialist services in 2008; almost three quarters
were completely satisfied with the primary care they received (www.NHSSurveys.
org/publications). But not all care is of high quality. There is plenty still to be
done to ensure that resource pressures and organisational arrangements do not
undermine good care, and that there is a culture in which staff remain motivated,
alert to the needs and expectations of those who use their services, are able to
keep up to date, and ready to improve. As this chapter was being written, late in
2011, the final report of the enquiry into standards of care at Mid Staffordshire
Trust was awaited. Both the Patients' Association (2011a, 2011b) and the Equality
and Human Rights Commission (2011) published reports deeply critical of the
standards of care and of the failure to afford human dignity to patients in hospital.

High quality care for all (Department of Health, 2008) was the title of the final
report from Lord Darzi, when Parliamentary Secretary of State at the Department
of Health. It was the result of a wide-ranging consultation. He concluded that
the NHS in England should be much more firmly aligned around quality, with
systematic measures and routinely published performance data, and that continuous
improvement should be properly recognised and rewarded. The government
responded with a National Quality Board, among other things, bringing together
stakeholders, lay and expert, to help realise the vision.

It is still early days. But will more central agencies, more measures, more advice,
more toolkits and guides help the situation? It is hard to argue that rankings

and ratings should go – but it is equally hard to argue that they guarantee better results. Darzi acknowledged staff frustration. A common refrain among clinicians and service managers continues to be that that they spend so much time feeding the machine – reporting on targets for the Department of Health and providing frequently changing information for regulators – that this crowds out the reviews of their own work that they want to do. Significantly, the innovations discussed by contributors to this section are bottom–up rather than top–down.

Much has been written over the years on defining and measuring quality. A simple but powerful maxim is that quality is doing the right thing at the right time in the right way. What this actually means in healthcare is suggested in the following box.

Quality is doing the right thing, at the right time, in the right way

Giving high-quality healthcare means:

- Attending to the safety of the patient at all times.
- Respecting the dignity and capabilities of patients throughout their care.
- Being aware of the relevant guidelines and the most recent evidence of effectiveness.
- Involving patents wherever possible in decisions about their own care.
- Applying up-to-date knowledge in the light of the patient's context and circumstances to achieve the best possible clinical outcome.
- Working together with other members of the care team to achieve the best possible result.
- Engaging with information on costs and with the potential for value-for-money savings.
- Reviewing information on your practice and on patient experience of it on a regular basis.
- Getting involved in service improvements that link your work with the overall patient experience of a journey through care.

Quality from a patient's point of view

The first three contributors to this section all focus in a highly practical way on the experience of quality. Jan Walmsley takes the tail end of a care episode she experienced. She had had successful cataract surgery. Those final checks were important for safety and for achieving the best possible clinical outcome. But could the right thing be achieved with less frustration and with less cost? She certainly has ideas worth considering. And there is a wider point. Cataract operations have transformed the lives of older people compared with those of earlier generations. How many other post-operative visits can be done closer to home – in local health clinics, or perhaps by telecare (Bunt and Harris, 2009)? There are other high-volume healthcare interventions that could be considered – all necessary if we are to remain paid workers not pensioners up until our late sixties and beyond.

Dignity is the focus of Catherine Dale's inspiring service redesign story of how a small change can make a big difference in the care experience of breast cancer patients. Hers is a vivid demonstration of the lesson of providing the right kind of forum – one that will engage with patients as partners and encourage them into speech can be a real eye-opener for practitioners and service managers alike. The concerns patients have are not always what staff expect. It can be a real surprise to staff when patients bring not just problems, but solutions – ones that make for a more rewarding experience all round. There are now many such service redesign projects, making a wide array of changes, improving the flow of patients and information through the system, and contributing to the well-being of patients and staff alike. Yet speeding improvements into usual practice right across the NHS remains a challenge – as the cataract care example demonstrated.

Much ink has been spilled on the topic of commissioning services in recent years and much more is about to be used as clinical commissioning groups get under way. A key argument has been that clinicians are closest to patients. But will they be more likely do the right thing? Will they engage directly with service users? Georgina Craig turns attention to what seems a particularly challenging case – commissioning end-of-life care. Craig found patients who were willing and, indeed, eager to give a point of view and brought recorded interviews to the commissioning table. Interestingly, for health workers, the patient on the screen or the recorded voice can sometimes be heard more readily than the patient in the room. The well-established work of Heath Talk Online (www. healthtalkonline.org) and the more recent Patient Stories (www.patientstories. org.uk) bear witness to this. Craig's topic was end-of-life care – but it could just as easily be commissioning, for example, for preventive services and public health.

The common thread in all these contributions, however, is that staff checking out issues from a service-user perspective can unfreeze thinking and bring fresh ideas, better practices for patients and, as Dale's account shows, a renewed sense of commitment from the staff. Another simple, direct and totally inspirational example of this can be found in the leadership section of this book, in the contribution by Willis. So why is it that change is slow? John Worth offers an answer to do with a deeply embedded culture in the NHS that unthinkingly disempowers service users. He knows full well that some readers will be reluctant to think that there are lessons from customer care in Apple and John Lewis – but his analysis certainly challenges us to get back to the fundamentals of what quality care should mean.

Quality as the reduction of human error

Patient safety has exploded onto the health policy agenda in recent years with the arrival (and reorganisations), for example, of a National Clinical Assessment Service and a National Patient Safety Agency and rapidly growing bodies of research. Important lessons have been learned from other industries, for example, about designing out error (in drug packaging), or using double-checking paperwork (in operating theatres). But these mechanisms, together with appraisals, continuing professional development and revalidation, important as they are, can never entirely eliminate human error. The next two contributors, both doctors, know this and urge owning up to mistakes and learning from them.

Tim Craft, a medical director, puts a harrowing story of surgical failure in paediatrics to positive use in persuading colleagues of the value of devising and following protocols about the safe introduction of new procedures. Clinicians and managers are understandably wary of the potential for litigation and the costs of compensation for those whose lives are permanently affected by the mistakes of the NHS. An organisation like Action Against Medical Accidents (www.avma. org.uk) alone deals with several thousand people in a year. It is notable, however, that in the case Craft describes, the mother of Beth has welcomed the use of her story to teach clinicians – an activity, indeed, in which she herself has taken an active part. Creating and maintaining quality care requires sensitivity, humility, honesty and above all courage from all who are involved.

Rick Stern has a similar message in a different context. Individual failures are often also system failures and failures to create, as he puts it, 'a culture and ethos that puts patient safety first'. His story of an avoidable death in an out-of-hours GP service graphically portrays the defensiveness of those concerned and the tendency to focus on money matters more than on good care. The initiative he describes is a response that acknowledges the human factor. It creates an accessible and safe space for service providers to contribute incidents and to learn from mistakes. Patients do tend to paint doctors larger than life – something like this gives clinicians a chance to admit that they do sometimes get it wrong. Stern mentions leadership – taken up in the final section of this book; his message is also about devising systems to support not just doctors, but all staff, to do the right thing.

Being open to service redesign and learning from error help to give meaning to the components of quality outlined earlier in this overview. Seeking improvements in quality needs to be part and parcel of professional behaviour. Stephen Dorrell MP, a previous Health Secretary, has been particularly outspoken on the matter. Introducing annual Health Committee reports on the regulators on 26 July 2011, he spoke of 'true professionalism' as involving intolerance of the second best: 'It is this intolerance which is the best safeguard of the standards of care delivered to patients' (see: www.parliament.uk). Speaking more informally at a conference at around the same time, he referred to 'divine discontent' as a quality all professionals should cultivate.

A quality health service for a local community

But if quality has to come above all from the competence and the commitment of all those delivering care, it must also come from the same attributes among those managing, supporting and leading the care. The quality of services on offer has to be everyone's business, and must permeate the system as a whole. This is where David Nicholson's 'third phase' (mentioned in the opening quotation) comes in: 'bringing it all together'. And this is also where the final contribution in this section is particularly relevant.

Catherine Foot offers us a valuable glimpse of a much larger piece of work that has been monitoring what happened when the government insisted that health trusts in England bring it all together by producing accessible 'quality accounts' for their local communities. Few found it easy. She directs a number of important messages to those charged with producing such accounts – reminding them, for example, to write for the intended readership, to explain and to be honest about what has worked and what has not. Why is it such a struggle to write about the achievement of quality? We can perhaps link this with a point made at the outset of this overview – high-quality healthcare is something that all too often occurs despite the systems of information management and use that are in operation, rather than *because of* them. In other words, the heath service does not seem to be *governed* in a way that is conducive to quality.

Governance is about 'the oversight and balancing of financial, clinical and patient satisfaction objectives' (Storey et al, 2011, p 3). Some would go further. The Good Governance Institute has brought the influential work on corporate governance in South Africa by Mervyn King to the attention of the NHS (Bullivant and Corbett-Nolan, 2011). King suggests that a report on the performance of any company and, indeed, of any corporate body should be 'a three-legged stool' with commercial, environmental and societal outcomes. Given the massive impact international companies have on the well-being of people and of the planet, he argues that 'integrated reporting' on these three elements is what we should expect. Local quality accounts for the NHS in England have some way to go before this kind of thinking is fully embedded. More inclusive forms of governance (discussed in Section Three) may well help with this.

Whether one works with a broader or narrower definition of governance, there is a key role for management boards and senior managers in the business of 'bringing it all together'. Boards are at the interface between service providers and service users in a locality. They need to develop a deep understanding of the range of services that are and are not on offer in their patch. They need to know the local demographics and to be in touch with health inequalities and community concerns. They need to appreciate the opportunities and constraints provided by wider policy developments. And, with all this in mind, they need to be able to tease out the meanings of the indicators and measures of quality in the different kinds of reports that they receive. As boundary-spanners they can play an important part in anticipating reactions, spotting potential misunderstandings and sometimes offering thinking outside the box. Storey et al (2011) usefully pull together and develop advice and guidance on how boards can work more effectively.

There is an elephant in the room and it is now starting to make an appearance. Improvements in health and healthcare to date have been achieved in times of growth. The NHS, along with other public services, now faces the challenge of doing more with less. In this context, as many observers are now saying, the challenge cannot simply be about maintaining quality at lower cost, but must involve innovations in the 'What?' and the 'How?' of healthcare. As Section One has also argued, this is particularly important both in tackling long-term conditions and in tackling the health challenges of modernity – obesity, drug and alcohol misuse, depression, and anxiety, for example. One helpful strand of work comes from the think-tank NESTA with its programme of work under the rubric of radical efficiency (Bunt and Harris, 2009; Gillinson et al, 2011). Radical efficiency means different services with lower costs and better outcomes for service users. Using bottom-up approaches, they make claims for cost savings that in some cases are very substantial indeed. Yet, these authors are able to draw from work across public services and from innovative companies such as Virgin and Orange; they use international as well as national examples. They stress that centrally enforced efficiencies are limited in their impact (Bunt and Harris, 2009, p 10) and are convinced that open innovation that gives power to front-line staff, patients and the public is the way to make radical changes widespread. Their underpinning concept of 'people-powered public services' is one that chimes well with contributions in this and other sections of this book and will be revisited in the final chapter.

Whatever one thinks about the 'fantastic journey' described by Sir David Nicholson at the head of this chapter, the alignment around quality called for by Lord Darzi back in 2008 is not yet firmly in place. The strong commitment to quality among those working in the NHS was clear when that report was being prepared. The practical actions described in this section more than demonstrate that those working on the front line are seizing opportunities where they can to make improvements. The main message of the contributors, however, is just how much value there is in working directly with patients on the quality improvement agenda, and harnessing for the NHS the free good they can offer – their reminders of what matters and their ideas about improvement of care. This is a theme taken up in the next section, where we look more directly at questions of governance.

SECTION 3

Governance – how can we really work together?

Introduction

The direct participation of ordinary people – as service users and as citizens – in the planning and provision of public services is embedded in legislation and is the subject of much guidance in the fields of health and social care. But a 'must do' is not always a 'can do' or even a 'want to do'. Until we understand – with examples – the benefits that can come from more inclusive governance of services, and until we have the competences to make a reality of that inclusion, accusations of cosmetic change, lip service, tokenism and box-ticking will continue.

David Sines offers a glimpse of what the benefits might be. Back in the early stages of his career as a nurse manager in learning difficulties, he worked with a patient advocacy organisation. The result changed him and changed the lives of the people with whom he was working. **Rohhss Chapman** and **Lou Townson** come up to date with an inspiring example of what can be achieved when people with learning difficulties are directly involved in researching services and contributing to change. Theirs is a fine response to any who would doubt the capacities and capabilities of a service-user group. What, then, if service users step into the system rather than working outside it? **Kate Ansell** gives a vivid account of how it feels to be the sole patient representative – the stranger in the room, bewildered and bemused by ways of working in the health sphere. Her work reminds us that simply bringing service users and service providers together is no guarantee of making the changes that will make a difference. **Beryl Furr** follows this with another inspiring account of what can be done. With the right training and support, ordinary citizens can be part of the service transformations we need – transforming themselves along the way. **Jane Keep** pulls together some of the secrets of successfully working with citizens and service users. A seasoned facilitator, she is aware of what those in the NHS are likely to take for granted, and she offers new ways of thinking and acting that can make all the difference.

A veritable 'patient and public engagement (PPE) industry' has grown up over the last decade or so in local government and in health, with its experts and advisors, but is it helping? **David Gilbert**, acknowledging his own place in that industry, writes a deliberately provocative piece that raises some important doubts. Finally, editor **Celia Davies** reflects on the various contributions and sifts through some recent academic writing on citizen and service-user engagement. Local community forums, patient panels, reference groups and so on are places, she says, where different worlds collide. To admit the unease that this creates is to start to identify what needs to be done to create more innovative, rewarding and constructive exchanges about just how health and well-being can be improved.

16

Reminiscences of an advocate

David Sines

It was over 30 years ago, in January 1979, that I was appointed to the post of Community Nursing Officer for people with a learning disability for the London Boroughs of Kingston and Richmond upon Thames. This was in the wake of what must be described as one of the very worst government inquiries in the history of learning disability care – the Normansfield Hospital Inquiry. Community care was still at a point of genesis, and reliance on hospitals such as Normansfield was the norm with regard to the care of people with learning disabilities.

At the heart of the new community care philosophy adopted at that time was the focus placed on the service user. We were ably assisted in our task of developing a client-oriented service through work undertaken by a notable activist and facilitator, Bob Sang, who had been appointed to work with an organisation called Advocacy Alliance. Advocacy Alliance was comprised of a band of dedicated volunteers who aspired to break through the bastions of control that resided within the institutions by empowering service users and speaking up on their behalf. The willing volunteer advocates at my first meeting with Advocacy Alliance included the then notorious *Times* newspaper columnist and critic, Bernard Levin, and a range of other celebrities, entrepreneurs and their supporters. Normansfield had provided a home for at least one TV celebrity's offspring, and, as such, enjoyed the patronage of members of the Variety Club of Great Britain who had the foresight to try to 'normalise' life opportunities for people in the hospital. The provision of independent advocacy was a critical ingredient in our aspiration to enrich the lives of those residents at Normansfield that were fortunate enough to be assigned such supporters. It opened up new opportunities for their stories to be heard and shared without fear of recrimination both within and outside hospital at that time.

During the five years that I worked with Advocacy Alliance, I learned to integrate the professional skills I had acquired during my university-based nurse education with the human skills that our volunteer advocates so generously shared with all persons with whom they worked. We were successful in introducing a range of new developments and life experiences that were quite unheard of at that time: for example, opportunities were extended to a number of residents to vote, to engage in regular shopping expeditions to the nearby boutiques and department stores of Kingston upon Thames, to enjoy meals in restaurants, to discover lost relatives, and to have access to their own money, thus allowing chances for the pursuit of personal ambitions.

Perhaps one of the greatest lessons learned was the need to listen attentively to a range of different opinions and to cultivate a genuine commitment among members of the professional care team to recognise the individuality of service users and their rights to share regular experiences in the form of narrative and dialogue. As a result, care plans began to change from rhetorical professional accounts to a series of person-centred aspirational life plans, populated with 'wish lists', many of which were realised through our combined teams' endeavours. We soon discovered that our objective should be to increase the amount of control that people with learning difficulties had over their lives, thus enhancing their sense of identity and increasing the range of opportunities for inclusion in the local community. Person-centred planning provided an effective vehicle through which to assist individuals to define, communicate and work towards achieving their life goals, in the context of family and other social networks and in a climate in which high expectations became the norm.

One other example of service change resulting from engagement with this model was that of the co-production of new service solutions – for example, brokering access for people with learning difficulties into ordinary services, such as further education colleges and primary healthcare services (rather than requiring them to continue to be dependent on attendance at social service day centres, special schools and segregated health services). We encouraged people to engage in mainstream life activities, using services alongside fellow citizens, with additional support where necessary. In turn, it meant that the rights of people with learning difficulties, for example, in relation to education, social services, employment, housing, transport and health, should be reflected in mainstream initiatives in each of these sectors and that barriers to inclusion should be challenged and if possible removed.

I shall never forget my days at Normansfield and the many tacit learning experiences that I encountered during these formative stages of my career. This inspired me to develop my own interest in the field of learning disability and in the promotion and enhancement of human rights for this group of people.

17

Researching together – pooling ideas, strengths and experiences

Rohhss Chapman and Lou Townson

This chapter is about the collaborative working of the Carlisle People First Research Team. There are currently eight of us and we act as a cooperative. We have been working together on research since 1998, although some of us have worked together in developing advocacy since 1990. We are a mixture of people: experts by experience who are labelled with learning difficulties, academic researchers and advocacy workers. However, these divisions are superficial; what matters is that we are all really interested in research and have chosen to be in the team.

The research team began when, in our advocacy roles, we were asked to gather people's views at an adult training centre that was closing down. When we arrived, it became clear that the people at the adult training centre had no idea that they were moving out; they did not know what we were asking them about. We were unhappy with this and felt a little used. We delayed the project until management did their work of informing people as to what was happening. Only then did we go back and start to collect their views. To our minds, there were a lot of things wrong about this process. It was about asking people how they felt after major decisions had been made, rather than using their views to shape what could happen. However, we reflected that this type of research work could be very useful in a wider sense to people with learning difficulties. We began to discuss what research was and to build our ideas around how projects could be useful for people.

After this experience, we formed a separate team dedicated to research. We decided to work as a cooperative because we felt we all had things to offer. We developed an accessible *research cycle*, which we now use to guide all of our projects. We also have a *set of rules* or guidelines. These help us make sure that we are working in the way we all agree is best. We work from people's own experiences and then link this with the literature, and what has already been said and done about research by disabled people. We have learned together about different research skills, much of which has been based on experiential learning.

We follow the principles of emancipatory research as articulated by disabled academics, emphasising as a starting point that ideas for research projects should come from people with learning difficulties. We decided to gather the histories of people with learning difficulties and to look at their achievements (Eardley,

2001; Townson, 2004). We designed a project to record the wartime memories of people with learning difficulties in Cumbria (Dias et al, 2012). For this, we raised money from the Heritage Lottery Fund, employed co-researchers with and without learning difficulties, and paid them on the same scale. There were some interesting findings from this project, which can be found at a web-based exhibition (see: www.peoplefirstcumbria.co.uk/resources/research). We also started to support other people in writing about their experiences of self-advocacy, and published chapters about this in other books (Spedding et al, 2002; Docherty et al, 2006).

In addition to the accessible tools mentioned earlier, we adapt and use the 'PATH process', which is large and graphic and helps everyone to have a say (Sanderson et al, 1997). Another example is our *river of history*, a diagram that helped us to think through the setting up of People First groups when we were doing a project on self-advocacy in the UK. The image of this shows tributaries and rapids representing support and problems. It includes a 'time machine' for people to sit in and recover their life histories.

The river of history

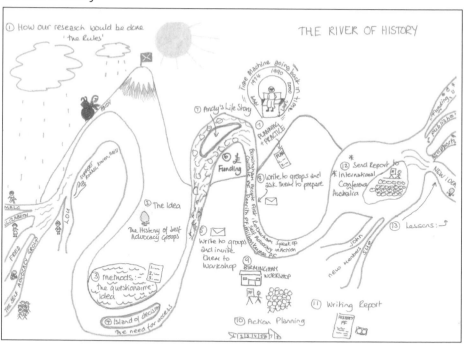

One of our guidelines is that our research has to involve people with learning difficulties in all stages of the research cycle. It was Elizabeth who came up with the idea that anywhere people were not included, they were actually being rejected. Everyone brings different strengths to the research team. Some can read and will feed the information back to others. We use plain language, videos and DVDs and invite 'expert' people to speak to us when seeking background information for projects. This wholly inclusive approach is more time-consuming but also adds value.

For example, during an interview, people with learning difficulties have at times been more open with peer researchers. Analysing findings together has allowed us to consider a range of interpretations based on people's own experiences; Andy put forward that a particular building was a possible safety hazard to wheelchair users, due to having encountered problems. Malcolm noticed who had been answering phones and raised the issue that some members were very shy. There are other examples of raised sensitivity to inaccessible paperwork, jargon, commands and noticing where people are spoken to differently.

A project that illustrates this holistic process well is the 'Self-advocacy and autism' project. The idea came from Elizabeth, who herself has a diagnosis of autism. She questioned how people on the autism spectrum could access advocacy if they did not like to attend group meetings. We agreed that this was an interesting question. Awards for All gave us backing for a pilot project in the north-west of England.

We started by finding out what other people had already said about the topic. Malcolm went to the local library and brought back books and videos. We watched the videos and discussed what we had seen. Lou and Rohhss took the books, read them and presented the information back for discussion.

As the fieldwork got under way, we attended self-advocacy meetings as observers and interviewed delegates at a conference led by people with autism. We ran a workshop and focus group for people with autism. Everyone took part in the fieldwork in the way they wanted.

After the information was collected, it was analysed by the team discussing the material together and identifying themes using large graphics stuck around the walls. We discovered that people found it difficult to fit in with the advocacy already available because it was not designed around their specific needs. We also found a lot of people commenting on their feelings of estrangement and 'not belonging'. We presented this at a conference and had the work published in the journal *Disability and Society* (Townson et al, 2007).

For us, the process of writing is about discussing the project while taping everyone's thoughts about it. The sentences are written up and we keep adding to them through group questioning until we agree on the final product. This can take a long time, but fits with our rule that we have to get our work into the public domain so that it can be useful to other people.

Analysis is sometimes said to be a difficult area for people with learning difficulties to be involved in. On a project about support workers, we used a method where the group worked out 'hypotheses' based on an analysis of what had been said about support at planning meetings. Later, we checked the findings against the hypotheses. These had included statements such as 'people with learning difficulties are not believed' and 'people's issues are swept under the carpet'. We set out to disprove or prove these points against instances of our observations and interviews.

Research takes place within the experience of our relationships in working together. Sometimes, when we are away on fieldwork, people may hear bad news from home or become ill or need help with personal issues. This can happen to any one of us, and each of us can assist each other. We feel that dividing people by labels does not reflect the complexity of our relationships.

We have met with resistance; sometimes people do not believe that people with learning difficulties can conduct good research. We have been asked to put our name to other people's projects so that they can demonstrate that they have been 'inclusive' where they had already decided what the project was and have only wanted token involvement. At the adult training centre, we were unknowingly put in a position of breaking bad news.

We have also faced problems with people who try to stop members being involved. One person had put his name forward for an international conference. A member of his staff went round to Rohhss's home and insisted that it was a bad mistake, shouting that he would never be able to manage and asking "How could you put these ideas into his head?". We all went abroad anyway and this member spoke fondly about his experiences for years afterwards. Most issues have been about people's attitudes and values rather than anything to do with our actual work. If we had responded to people who doubted us, we would never have got anywhere.

On the other hand, we have a good record for obtaining funding for projects, have written up our findings and had them published. We have presented our research at conferences at home and abroad. In doing so, we have met and have been indebted to a number of academics and people with learning difficulties, especially through The Open University's social history of learning disabilities group, who have connected us into their networks throughout the world.

Overall, we believe that anyone can work together collaboratively as long as they work at listening to and learning from each other. It is about the investment of time. Researching in this way not only benefits the people who are involved, but leads to better outcomes and ultimately does a little bit to improve the lives of people with learning difficulties.

18

Becoming accepted

Kate Ansell

> Patients, of course, have roles assigned to them within the scripts of the modern medical drama. Depending on who is doing the analysis or the accountancy, patients appear as demand, costs, benefits, input or output, voters, clients or consumers of services, bearers of rights or pursuers of litigation, the 'tib and fib' in bed 15, frozen sperm in the deep freeze, diseased bodies or clinical material, points on a graph or numbers crunched on a software programme. (Porter, 1997, p 668)

Sadly, there is still no universal recognition of the value and worth of the patient voice: that they are willing and able to contribute to discussions, have views that are worth listening to, or suggestions that might make a difference. Being involved is a challenge, becoming accepted is a bigger one.

But finding a way in may be easier said than done. There are plenty of invitations, usually posters on a noticeboard, asking if you have a few hours to spare or would like to be a member of a committee, with the sweeping invitation 'come along and join us' – but there is never anything to tell you what you are letting yourself in for. So how do you find out? You don't. Just jump in at the deep end and you will never regret it. The rewards are tremendous and, remember, you can always change your mind. That is a patients' choice.

So why are you getting involved? You thought it would be a way to say thank you for care received; you have learned to live with your condition and you want to help others to do the same; and, very occasionally, you want to find a way to share a bad experience with those who make the decisions, which might improve things for other patients.

Now the surprises begin. Your welcome to a meeting can take several forms. You can be treated with enthusiasm and bonhomie, or polite indifference. Either way the introductions round the table take place at such speed that you do not have a chance to write them down, let alone remember them. Mind you, rarely do job titles give you a clue of the actual job role. You can only sit there and hope that all will become clear.

Your first meeting will be the sharpest learning curve of all. You probably won't remember much of the work of the meeting because you will be fascinated by the procedures, or lack of them, as the chairman struggles to keep the meeting going forward. The apologies are confusion themselves: "She couldn't attend",

"He's come instead", "But they only work in the same office so he is not familiar with …". Another is on holiday and when they come back they are moving post and aren't being replaced. There are those who have to leave early and, so they can, want to jump to item eight on the agenda because they "have some exciting news" – a view that no one else seems to share. There are further disruptions by late arrivals who ask to be updated; those who are so busy tapping away on their blackberries or laptops that you wonder why they are there; and, horror of horrors, the one (and there is always one) who has another meeting to go to and "will miss lunch", so crunches noisily through a heap of carrots and celery.

Like everything, the first time is the worst. The first time you ask a question in a meeting be prepared for wide eyes all round the table, some audible tutting, some ceiling-gazing, and looks of horror – a patient who speaks – so much so that you wonder if you have developed a second head or, worse, that you are in the wrong meeting.

But it is going to get better, don't give up now, you have taken the most difficult step. Keep reminding yourself why you are there – you remember, you felt you had something to give, to try to make things better for other patients, to speak up for those who do not or who feel unable to do so, to put the patient view when changes or proposals are the topic, which you will often see very differently from the healthcare professionals sitting round the table with you. Never allow yourself to think of the enormity of the task that faces you – getting the NHS to listen to the patient voice.

The settling-in process is as interesting as the first meeting. You will quickly realise that however long the study group, task force or project development initiative has been in existence, the culture of the arrival of new faces whose roles might or might not be appropriate or applicable continues. But take heart; although they all work in the NHS, don't assume that they will all know each other, they won't, so you are not alone in not knowing who is who. Just sit quietly and watch.

As people arrive, they will form little clusters who have hushed conversations, sometimes casting a glance towards another group. The body language may be difficult to interpret but the snippets of the whispers are an insight: "How did he get selected for that post, he's only …?", "What is she doing here …?", "Why do they all have to come to every meeting, no wonder the department is in a mess?". For sure, it will be some perceived iniquity either of person, job or job role. But beware of overhearing the rhetorical question: "Whoever made the decision to move long term conditions to end of life?". Don't be tempted to put your hand up or say anything. You might be mistaken for management. Mind you, when the looks become directed towards you, you know that you are on the way to becoming accepted. They have noticed you, whether for good reasons or bad, it matters not which because you've done something that warrants comment. Worry not when you are told that "You didn't get it quite right", because you've achieved something that many a senior clinician or manager strives for without success – you've got the meeting talking!

Do not misread tentative approaches towards you. The caution is because they are having a patient experience of a different kind. You are not in the surgery, in the clinic or in a bed, needing care, medication or an operation; you are taking part in perfectly normal, well, national health conversations and joining in discussions. Each will have their own way of welcoming you into the fold, though mostly it will seemingly be to offload their filing cabinet of reports and papers that "you need to read". I promise you it is well intentioned and not a way of making sure you are soaked to oblivion in information, but a genuine wish to help you to become familiarised. Best way to deal with it: file it, get to know the task at hand in your own way.

Another step forward can be when someone suggests you give them a call to talk about the task at hand. However, doing as suggested, getting in touch, is not that simple when up against the patterns of the working week in the NHS. The combinations are fascinating, Monday, Wednesday and Friday; Monday, Tuesday and Friday – the three-day weeks. The five-day weeks are either at meetings or probably filling the gaps of the "No, I'm not in tomorrow" brigade. Add to the confusion those who work from home (Why? Is there a shortage of desks as well as beds in the NHS?) But the cracker is the Thursday girl who works Tuesday, Wednesday and Thursday and only responds to emails just before close of play on Thursday, and, of course, repeats the pattern the next week. Think about it, you can wait a fortnight for a reply to your query if she has a meeting on a Thursday!

Your next task is to find a way to take an active part, to get the team to let you work with them, to contribute, to let you do more than just sit in meetings, lending your voice occasionally. Asking the question "Is there a job for me?" usually brings a reply, as it did for me, of "Do you have the time?". Why do they think you are there! No, you have to ask a different question, be inventive. Is the project one where a patient view might be helpful? Is there an opportunity for you to give real examples of good or bad working, to put another slant on considerations? That is what you are there for, so you could suggest that a patient view might be helpful. You will probably be faced with an array of blank looks, many tinged with fear, but don't let that put you off. Find a pen and paper without delay.

But you still have to be patient, don't try to rush the last few steps to becoming accepted. When times are tough, always remind yourself that you didn't choose to be a service user, but you did choose to be a patient representative.

So go along to the meetings, the workshops, the conferences and enjoy yourself, ignore the fact that you will, at first, be regarded with suspicion, after all you are a patient, so how will you know anything about the NHS? They will soon find out!

19

Supporting 'experts by experience' – a champion idea

Beryl Furr

> Go to the people.
> Live amongst them.
> Start with what they have.
> Build with them.
> And when the deed is done,
> The mission accomplished,
> Of the best leadership,
> The people will say,
> 'We have done it ourselves'.

> (Widely attributed to Lao Tzu, *The Tao of Leadership*, various editions and various translations)

Just about every NHS reform since 1974 has introduced a new patient and public organisation. But structures and organisations count for nothing unless commissioners, providers and users share the realities of the NHS and how to achieve the mutual goal of safe, high-quality, cost-effective services in the face of structural reform, rising costs, increasing demand and the requirement to save £20bn by 2014/15.

Quality, Innovation, Productivity and Prevention (QIPP) is a case in point. Introduced in 2009, it is a wide-ranging initiative, bringing together representatives of local services, patients and the voluntary sector to improve quality and save costs by redesigning services that patients need, and reviewing options for services that people want (Department of Health, 2011). QIPP underlines the need to co-create a new vision for patient and public engagement (PPE) and to launch an open and honest discussion about what the Coalition government's promise – 'No decision about me, without me' (Department of Health, 2010a) – really means. It can only become a reality, however, if people understand how to share responsibility for health, not only at a personal level, but also at the wider level of resource use.

Educating for engagement

The aim of PPE is well understood by its practitioners, but remains a mystery to most of those who are engaged. However, as a facilitator, community activist, Community Health Council (CHC) chief officer and Primary Care Trust (PCT) non-executive director, I have had the privilege of working with patients and communities and being allowed to tap into the rich seam of humanity and creativity that people bring to engagement.

If people are to share the 'who, what, when and why', they must also know and trust the mechanisms for local accountability, understand why some needs are prioritised, what is possible and what is not, and know who to ask about 'Why not me?' and 'What will happen when the money runs out?' Strategists and policymakers also need confidence that the people who get engaged are reasonably well-informed and open-minded. We need more opportunities to learn together and teach one another how systems work, share stories and experiences about falling into 'gaps' and co-create innovative local solutions. How is this to be done?

Champions are doing it for themselves

'Creating community champions' in Southend-on-Sea ran from 2004 to 2007. Initially supported by an EU grant, a social enterprise – Chameleon Academy – launched and led the programme, offering a shared space to a mixed group of people from socially deprived communities, most with one or more long-term conditions. Invitations posted throughout the area invited those interested in becoming community champions (CCs) to sign up for the first 15-week course (and stay for lunch). In total, 110 people signed up for at least one of the four courses that made up the overall programme; 100 completed their chosen course and 60 people gained National Open College Network qualifications.

People brought their personal experience, curiosity, questions and ideas. They shared in developing the new knowledge and networks, skills and resources that would enable them to take control of their own health and well-being and engage their own families, neighbours and communities of interest. Learners co-created and presented the content and objectives of each course in partnership with tutors, health and social care practitioners, community and civic leaders, social entrepreneurs, actors, activists, artists, dance therapists, musicians and more.

Using a variety of techniques, groups practised how to navigate and influence local services, offer constructive challenges, be consulted, and consult others. 'Green' issues, project management, communication and media skills were some of the topics covered. Some stories needed to be heard by a wider audience, and a different group produced a video, *Listen to me*, on living with a mental health issue. Chairs, chief executives and senior officers accepted invitations to join facilitated conversations and 'tell it like it is': commissioning and providing services with limited resources, where the money goes, the complexities of assessing community needs and reaching consensus on whose could be met and whose not, and the implications of 'postcode' services. They spoke about the importance of building mutual trust and keeping that trust when plans were reduced or abandoned due to changing circumstances. They triggered a range of emotions from anger and frustration when the people in charge did not seem to 'get it', to fun and excitement when discussion sparked off new and different ways of doing things. The public leaders won respect for turning up – and for being honest.

Champion outcomes

People were full of ideas and enthusiasm – and ready to engage and choose their own outcomes. Some achieved their chosen level of National Open College Network qualifications, while others were happy just to become a resource for the community. Some 'graduates' became tutors on new courses created with mental health service users, young people 'Not in Employment, Education or Training' (NEETs) and community activists. Others developed the Southend Community Champions League: arranging social activities and sharing projects – from setting up a Time Bank to setting up charities (one of which replaced all 21 boats lost by a devastated Sri Lankan fishing community). Some formed a self-help group for families of children with attention deficit hyperactivity disorder (ADHD), and launched a 'Big Society Department Store' in 2011, offering affordable space to social entrepreneurs who are role models for the benefits and joys of doing things for themselves. All this emerged from people who were not natural 'joiners', who were amazed to find their own voices and who not only made them heard by 'the leaders', but became leaders themselves.

Programme outcomes were documented in an evaluation report by Lynette Adams, senior tutor for the programme, which can be found on the Academy website (www.chameleonacademy.co.uk). And while continued funding makes Chameleon's future precarious, a modified programme for adult community learning continues. Dilip Jesudasen, project director, and three champions (two of whom had never been outside England) travelled to Cyprus on one of two exchange projects, and hosted two events in Southend for partners from Holland, Germany, Denmark and Cyprus.

Why not me?

Rationing by ever-tighter criteria is increasingly common throughout the NHS. However, there are no 'blanket bans' and people may request a case review if they feel they can show that they are an exception to the rule. Some PCTs conduct paper exercises, but hearing directly from patients is an essential part of PPE. I chaired a panel that invited patients to talk with us before any decision was made about individual funding. We explained clearly and simply why the NHS could not fund everything and we were constantly humbled by people's grace and compassion for those with greater needs. We listened to painful stories about discomfort, embarrassment and failed efforts to help themselves. Even when we were obliged to say 'no', we could at least acknowledge their humanity, thank them and manage their expectations. It invariably deepened understanding on both sides, but people still had to live with their condition, and many felt let down by the NHS's denial of treatment for lifestyle-related conditions.

These patients are just the tip of the iceberg: the NHS cannot continue to meet the ever-increasing demand for services from finite resources. Further rationing and disillusionment is inevitable as more and more people are required to accept greater personal responsibility for health and the use of NHS resources. But some of those resources could be invested in developing the capacity of people to understand 'Why not me?' and how to help themselves and those around them. Let us turn 'Why not me?' into 'How can I learn to deal with this?' or 'How can we work together to help ourselves?'

Despite illness or disability, people are never just a patient or carer, but are always human. Every life has overlapping and interconnecting needs, aspirations and expectations. If the NHS fails to meet, or sometimes when it exceeds, those expectations, it can trigger a crisis, leading people to form a close relationship with a specific service because they want to help to improve services following a complaint, or to 'give something back'. These very humane responses can make a huge contribution to the continuous cycle of improvement. However, having invested energy and emotion, people resist proposals to close, shift or replace 'their' service, and they may take to the barricades to save it. If the local MP is standing by, it is usually with one eye on the next election and the other on the microphone, but it is a rare MP who speaks up for modernisation, greater efficiency or makes a case for the wider community of patients. We need honesty and plain-speaking about what services are necessary and possible, and the part that people need to play in them.

For the future

Everybody is different, and people want engagement that suits their needs, time and temperament. Most contribute and move on – completing questionnaires or surveys, posting a card in the suggestion box, speaking to PALS, or making a complaint. Others join self-help groups or Practice Participation Groups. But, however they choose to engage, few people begin with a clear idea of what is involved. Professionals also need to acknowledge when they are out of their depth and seek help on how, when and where to provide support.

The NHS needs resourceful communities who can tackle their own inequalities and help to create the health and well-being solutions that they want and will use. The Southend programme was created with and for local people, but a number of others promoting community learning and community action have been developed throughout the country (see the box regarding NIACE and the Yorkshire and Humberside health champions project at the end of this chapter). Creating community champions could be a real investment in PPE as well as a real help to the NHS.

Want to know more about creating community champions?

- NIACE community learning champions support programme. Available at:
  www.niace.org.uk/current-work/community-learning-champions
- Yorkshire and Humberside health champions project – AltogetherBetter website. Available at:
  www.altogetherbetter.org.uk/community-health-champions
- Chameleon Academy website. Available at:
  www.chameleonacademy.co.uk

20

Engaging communities – sharing the learning

Jane Keep

Introduction

Primary Care Trusts were formed around a decade ago. A national primary and care trust development programme (NatPaCT) was created to support them in delivering their key objectives. Building their skills, knowledge and confidence in engaging communities was one key objective and, for this reason, the Engaging Communities Learning Network (ECLN) was created. In operation from between 2002 and 2005, this learning network drew in policy advisors, academics, patient and public involvement organisations, voluntary sector organisations, and patients themselves. It involved almost every Primary Care Trust in the country. This contribution highlights some of the key lessons about the building blocks of engagement. They are as relevant now as they were then.

Moving from extracting information to changing relationships

There is a big difference between methods of 'involvement' that are designed to extract information (surveys, polls, etc) and interventions that result in people and their relationships changing, such as community forums and citizens' juries (Stewart, 1996). In order to change, people need to be challenged emotionally and intellectually in a process of willing engagement in something new. As people engage with each other, so relationships change and, ultimately, so do behaviours and cultures. Our experience in the ECLN was that much so-called engagement was focused on extracting information rather than truly building relationships. Building relationships enables a deeper cultural change, and it takes more time than simply extracting information. What builds the relationship is a variety of interventions, most of which will be face-to-face over time, whereby those 'engaged' can build trust and feel that what is said and discussed is actually heard and acted upon.

Moving from using jargon to developing shared language

Removing 'NHS jargon' and finding a straightforward, common language is central to achieving meaningful mutual engagement. Language can create a barrier to clarity and understanding. We need to learn to 'bridge', so that we all have the possibility to come to a shared understanding. The way to do this requires common sense and a day-to-day practicality around the way we speak and what we speak about. When we are together, discussing and talking, we need to expose assumptions behind the words or statements, and to explore the meanings embedded in them. While this can take time, it reaps important benefits: the very process of exploring and explaining itself deepens our relationships with one another, as well as creating clarity in our understanding of what is being said, and why.

Anything that is not clear or expressed clearly can be gently challenged: if one person is not clear about it, then others will feel the same. Speaking up about what is not clear is also crucial to gaining shared meaning, and deepening our relationships together. When we hear things said that do not feel 'right' or clear, then we all have a responsibility to speak up and ask: 'Can you clarify that further?', 'Can you explain a bit more what you mean by that?', 'Is anything we are discussing based on assumptions we should explore?' and so on. This builds confidence in our expression with one another too.

Moving from reacting to responding

A shift can be made from reactive contributions or discussions, which can stem from fear or lack of understanding, towards enabling responsive contributions that demonstrate willingness (and the confidence) to involve and engage across the whole system. Enabling this shift is an often-needed behavioural change if communities are to effectively engage. Many of us can, at times, appear reactive rather than responsive to situations and to the feedback we receive. We can learn by developing our own self-awareness and self-observation, noting when we are reacting and when we are responding. Reactions are usually based on an emotional reaction to a given situation. Responses, by contrast, are considered and thought-through, where the speaker is clear on their own stance in the situation, and is seen to reflect on what is needed for the greater good in a given situation. Once we can role-model responding rather than reacting, others can be inspired to do the same.

When working together we are often aware when others are reacting rather than responding. We can learn to challenge this gently, so that working together becomes more focused on what is needed rather than the emotional needs of one individual. Modelling inclusive behaviour in this way is needed at all times, in virtual as well as 'live' events and forums, and both during backstage and front-stage work. This inclusivity promotes the realisation that we can all learn from each other, whatever our part in engaging or our role at work. Equally, co-creating new measures of success and benchmarking processes is something we can do together, rather than assuming that this must be done prior to a meeting. Engaging communities means creating cultures of participation, where everyone can be involved in everything – setting up, agreeing ground rules and principles for working together, agreeing processes of meetings and interventions, agreeing key questions that need addressing, agreeing the key success measures, and regularly reviewing how we are engaging with one another: 'Are we making a difference?'

Moving from the duty of partnership to co-governance and shared stewardship

True engagement requires moving from the 'duty of partnership' towards models of co-governance and shared stewardship. Often, there are no obvious models or tools, but these come by simply asking the questions when working together, such as: 'Are we merely acting from a duty of partnership, or are we open to co-developing co-governance or shared stewardship?'; 'What would the difference be practically, between acting from a duty of partnership and co-governance or shared stewardship?'; 'How would we know we had moved to shared stewardship, and what would be our success measures?'. This can feel difficult at times, but even the most difficult moments, shared and observed, can lead to greater development of trust and openness.

Using key questions to jointly review engaging processes

Some key questions are outlined in the following. They can be used in any part of a system by anyone, at any time, to help promote inclusiveness while working together. Questions like these could well be co-designed with all those with whom you are engaging:

- How much do you currently engage, and how participatory is it?
- How will you ensure engagement is co-developed with a shared ownership?
- Are there any participatory boundaries – is there anything that is not participatory?
- How do you jointly know you are truly participatory?
- How do you know your engagement and involvement is adding value?
- How do you jointly know the difference your interventions are making in a practical sense?
- What 'sticks'? What sustains? And so what is the 'glue' in your relationships when you engage?
- Who sets the success measures and who is involved in review?
- What assets do you already have and what can you build out from?
- What joint succession planning do you have or need if you are looking for sustainability in the longer term of your relationships and the engagement and inclusivity you have developed?

- Who are the brokers and buffers – for example, how do you help to quieten the political 'noise'?
- How will you jointly acknowledge, share and celebrate success?

To conclude ...

We know that working in a participatory, inclusive and engaging way provides a more systemic and sustainable way of doing things, whatever needs to be done. It initially simply requires an openness to the possibility that things can change, and a willingness to ask seemingly awkward questions, as well as try and test new ways of working together in a non-judgemental learning environment. All of this is possible, 'playfully'. Too often we are too serious and intense about these things, when naturally human beings like to work together playfully. Once we appreciate how much value working engagingly is, we can continue to build on this together. After all, it is not a one-off process, but a lifelong way of living and working together.

Want to know more about the 'engaging communities' learning?

- Cowper, A., Keep, J. and Sang, B. (2004) 'Opening our eyes to choice, risk and accountability', *British Journal of Healthcare Management*, vol 10, no 11, pp 329–33.
- Keep, J. and Sang, B. (2005) 'Engaging the intermediate tier in "a patient-led NHS"', *British Journal of Healthcare Management*, vol 11, no 7, pp 204–8.
- Keep, J. (2007) 'Making an impact through integrating learning methodologies – a large scale, collaborative, systems-based learning network in the British National Health Service', in S. Sambrook and J. Stewart (eds) *Human resource development in the public sector – the case of health and social care*, London: Routledge.

21

The engagement industry – some personal reflections

David Gilbert

[T]he involvement of 'lay' people in the NHS remains on the terms dictated by those within the system.... Health related organisations ... have become compromised instruments of 'co-management' of the NHS, accepting a place at the table in order to secure funding and recognition. (Sang, 2002, p 381)

How many of us really listened to – or want now to listen to – this critique of our merry band of engagement evangelists? Over recent years, the engagement industry has grown to encompass a disparate group: academics, policy wonks, methodological gurus, survey implementers, data-gatherers, equipment and kit suppliers, webmasters, advisers and consultants (like me), third-sector advocates, activists and representatives, the list could go on. Is all this activity a sign of an emerging social movement for change leading to improvements in responsiveness and accountability? Or have we been deluded by our frenetic activities into believing that processes equate to impact?

Have we become over-reliant on gathering data at the expense of clarity about purpose? Is it a mask that prevents dialogue between organisations and communities? Has a preoccupation with representational structures led to individuals 'going native' (the *modus operandi* of institutions)? Has a professional specialty arisen that serves to exclude front-line staff?

We have policies in place for patient and public engagement (PPE) like never before. We have regulators banging on the doors to ensure PPE compliance. Primary Care Trust (PCTs) (soon to be disbanded) climbed up the slippery pole of world-class commissioning, in part by improving their PPE activities. The Coalition government wants 'Nothing about me, without me'. Structures change, what matters to patients remains the same.

On 'our side', we have formal structures providing a statutory patient voice. In England, CHCs, PPI Forums and now LINks have come and gone. HealthWatch emerges. There is no end, rightly, to the clamour for accountability and responsiveness. A wealth of academic research into PPE is under way, knowledge of what works is on the rise. The NHS is awash with data from surveys and consultations – the phrase 'consultation fatigue' is well-rehearsed.

But I don't see universal buy-in to this agenda from senior leaders, clinicians and front-line staff. Nor is there a groundswell of exciting involvement opportunities – rather, a tired and clunky engagement industry reliant (in the main) on old-fashioned methods and archaic representative structures. Have we made much progress? Or has a castrated engagement industry grown up – one that is struggling to move beyond isolated (in the past, well-funded) projects? Meanwhile, innovative ideas (largely borrowed from other sectors), technological possibilities, a desperate desire for different ways of meeting unmet need – note the current fascination for social entrepreneurism and enterprise – and the idea of 'patients as leaders' emerge from the shadows.

Structures but ...

A recent workshop painted a picture of the 'representative structures': I have an experience of services, go to a user forum. A representative takes views to an advisory group, which takes these to some organisational (or partnership) subcommittee, which feeds into another committee, then to a senior management team and/or finally a Board. Each time the real meaning of the minutes taken at the original meeting, if taken at all, becomes diluted or distorted through a Chinese-whisper-like process.

Meanwhile, managers gather more evidence ('valid' and 'triangulated' data) about people's experience (through consultations, surveys and focus groups) and blend it (drown it?) with non-patient-derived data (routine or 'performance' data). The murky fog of finance, risk and governance intelligence descends. A 126-page set of agenda papers is taken to the Board in order for a decision to be made on next steps.

Finally, a policy declares an organisation to be 'patient-centred' (patient groups declare victory) and is (sort of) implemented via an equally obscure chain of command. Will my experience change the next time I am admitted to hospital? Was it worth me going to the user forum in the first place? The Board has been buffered from hearing my story, and the thousands of everyday experiences at the front line. Nothing changes. Of course, this is a caricature, but it will seem familiar to many.

We have become accustomed to feeding the beast. When a new set of institutional structures appears, engagement advocates clamour for a seat at the table. Formal structures are important but too often debate about purpose and function (of structures) and the role and skills (of the individual) becomes subservient to form. 'We' complain about 'them' doing 'tick-box' engagement, but inadvertently comply. All energies are on what happens in committees, little on the myriad informal mechanisms required for dialogue and building trusting relationships.

Moreover, the poorly equipped representative is stuffed – unable to get their voice heard, isolated among professional power-brokers, drowning in a sea of papers sent to them the day before, getting more and more red-faced in the corner. But woe betide them if they get angry. Further marginalisation awaits 'inappropriate behaviour' (a wonderfully useful term). They have to learn to play the game. Dissent quietens and an uneasy truce prevails, particularly if the representative is seduced and flattered (as I was) into accepting the *status quo*.

InHealth Associates runs learning programmes on 'the effective patient and community representative' and is both exploring the concept of patient leadership (Gilbert, 2012a, 2012b) and developing a Centre for Patient Leadership (www. inhealthassociates.co.uk). Might these sorts of initiatives unleash a new generation of patient leaders – activists, representatives, community health leaders or entrepreneurs – who will step up to the plate and find new ways of doing things?

Big events but ...

Years ago, a bus driver refused me and my sleeping baby in a pushchair access unless I folded it (the pushchair, not the baby). Later, I noticed a poster inviting me to 'have my say' at a consultation event on 'local integrated transport systems'. But it sounded like a turgid evening, and there was football on TV.... I know purposeful events are held all over the place, but those where data feeds into decision-making are the exception. Can we turn data-gathering exercises into smart ways of asking people (as experts) for solutions to tough problems? I know many friends brimming with ideas and passion to help. I would have given my views if I had been asked in the right place, in the right way, at the right time.

I don't see many front-line staff enthused by PPE. I know staff don't always 'know' what matters to patients. But by creating an engagement industry based on big set pieces or quantitative methods, we risk marginalising front-line staff and undervaluing their expertise. A recent project we carried out – '1000s of everyday conversations' – gave front-line staff post-it notes (the most expensive equipment we needed). We asked them to ask patients during the course of a consultation or at the front desk 'What one thing could we do better?'. They were to gather the ideas on the post-its so that we could come up with small but crucial interventions.

Research but ...

There is a lot of interesting academic research on PPE. But if you are a chief executive or GP commissioner, how long can you wait for the findings? As part of evaluating a fabulous peer-to-peer mental health mentoring scheme, we talked to commissioners about funding its roll-out. "Great idea," they said; but they could not take a punt on a 'non-proven' idea. We pointed to emerging qualitative work that suggested huge benefits. Not good enough. A risk-averse NHS had no room to innovate, despite a 25% rise in hospital admissions. The voluntary organisation piloting the idea had to get more money to generate the evidence that commissioners wanted – how the work impacts on admissions, prescribing and return to work. By the time they got the evidence, restructuring had taken place and relationships had fragmented.

Of course, research takes time. But the academic industry can be self-serving ('dissemination' equals citations in academic journals). Does the evidence generated by researchers address questions that commissioners and providers (and patients!) need? Or does it merely generate interesting debates between policy wonks and academics?

Now, within a cash-strapped system, we need to demonstrate (rightly) the benefits of PPE. There is some evidence that high-quality PPE can improve things. For example, a recent project with Frontline Consultancy for the Department of Health provided documented case studies of PPE at each stage of the commissioning cycle, which seemed to have significant economic benefits (Frontline and InHealth Associates, 2012). Meanwhile, Picker has undertaken work on the evidence for PPE (see: www.investinengagement.info). But can this be quickly translated into a business case for managers and GP commissioners who need persuasion that there is something in PPE for them (eg reducing workload)?

Meanwhile, leaders do not get the data for timely decisions, and local innovation gets crowded out and cannot compete in the 'evidence-based' evaluation stakes. Again, engagement fails to make an impact.

Projects but ...

We have excellent local engagement projects, often around service improvement, but this does not seem to translate into ensuring that we have patient-friendly, organisational culture and systems. Projects remain on the periphery, winning annual awards or gaining *Guardian* feature space.

We have got PPE toolkits coming out of our ears. The 'how' of engagement now means methodologies and techniques rather than practical support on influencing organisational change. Many agencies can run surveys or focus groups, but fewer can align this with organisational development, change management or leadership. Whizzy events leave participants happy until they realise that nothing much has changed at the coalface and that the report is still on the shelf.

Fresh (if that is the word) from my mental health experiences, I once went to a 'blue-sky' four-day event on local mental health services, where we held out for six local outreach services. The finance director came in on the final day and said that only one could be financed. If the facilitators had been honest about resources, we would have been frustrated, but appreciated it. The final afternoon was great, trying to help the finance director find a solution. It wasn't easy, talking about thresholds for inclusion into the scheme, but we trusted him due to his honesty.

Data but ...

There seems an increasing focus on data around quality and patient experience. Might this risk turning the rich world of engagement into a technocratic and desiccated exercise? Only dialogue and trusting relationships can provide the data to transform services. If people are treated as repositories of data, filling in ever-more questionnaires, inputting into thousands of hand-held devices, a new generation of informatics gurus will usurp PPE. Will it become easier for organisations to divorce themselves from 'shared decision-making'? Engagement practitioners, driven by their community roots, may become further marginalised as power resides elsewhere.

I once met a director for commissioning and asked how hospital survey data informed commissioning decisions. Her reply: "I don't have time to read them". She argued that she was patient-centred and would send a non-executive director to look at car parking and food quality (Wrong on so many levels!). I knew the issue was staff attitudes. Later, I saw a huge pile of surveys outside the public health directorate. There was no time to analyse them: "Something urgent has come up," said the junior analyst. Did she not see the data as important? She laughed: "I do, but others don't." How much money was wasted on an industrial amount of data leading to zero change?

Of course, there are online solutions – excellent ones that build in facilities for dialogue (see, eg, Hodgkin in Section 4). But I have seen managers ignore that material too, as it is at 'arm's length'. The urge for data destroys the potential for dialogue (Iles has something more to say on this; see Section 4). It is certainly easier to manage bits of data than share decisions with complex, passionate people.

Conclusion

We seem to have a frenzied engagement system that fails, on the whole, to engage leaders (managers, Boards), front-line staff (clinical and non-clinical) and patients and the public. The way it operates – big set pieces, projects, structures, research, data – seems to maintain the *status quo* rather than challenge it. Have we created an industry that is self-serving; one that produces minimal or unsurprising output, by co-opting people into, and taming data to fit, institutional structures? We can shift the structures as much as we like, but it won't change anything unless we find a new way of doing things.

22

Overview: Colliding worlds – the journey towards collaborative governance

Celia Davies

The explosion of activities over the last two decades in the NHS under the banner of public and patient involvement (PPI; later 'engagement', PPE) has parallels across all areas of public services. Pupil and parent participation in the operation of schools, participation of residents and service users in local authority areas, inviting citizens in at national public policy formation level, all of these and more have been part of a quest to improve services and make them more responsive to the needs of those they serve. But, as David Gilbert shows in this section, there is unease, even among the enthusiasts, and calls are being made for evidence about impact. This chapter brings into sharper focus some of the dilemmas discussed by the contributors to this section, underlining the importance both of new styles of interaction and new forms of organising.

Even with goodwill and commitment, a great deal can go wrong with initiatives to involve service users or the wider public – whether this is in the delivery of services or their overall design. Enthusiastic citizens, for example, often complain that they are bombarded with unintelligible documents, that nothing that occurs seems to relate to their motivation to join and that there seems to be no place in formal meetings to link their experience with the issues on the table. Kate Ansell remains positive about becoming accepted, but unfamiliar procedures and behaviours can drain outsider confidence, or lead to anger and cynicism. Managers and practitioners may also have doubts, fearing that service users will not understand the context of their work or will just use the opportunity to complain. On the one hand, they may be concerned that citizens will be disruptive, and, on the other, that they will be silent, intimidated in the face of expert debate.

These are some of the familiar experiences that occur when separate worlds collide. Take long-term conditions (see Section 1). These conditions represent identity-enhancing, specialist knowledge challenges for professionals. They are unwelcome spoilers of an identity for a care service user, whose reactions are likely to include denial and despair, perhaps a dogged inward-looking determination to cope, followed sometimes by a crusading zeal for service change. Public service managers and professionals, strongly committed to their fields, will have nonetheless acquired a degree of emotional detachment, which is important to the conduct of their daily work. Service users are most definitely not detached. The worlds of citizens are different again: community spirit, a sense of 'giving something back' or perhaps simply 'keeping active', tends to engage an older generation, whereas, for many, it can be a complaint not satisfactorily resolved that galvanises action. The rewards to be derived from service improvement may be similar all round, but without the payback of the pay-packet or career, motivations and expectations are just not the same.

The contributors to this section both exemplify these colliding worlds and offer some solutions to them. Ansell describes a deep gulf of understanding and practice when worlds collide. Chapman and Townson's answer is for a group of service users to do it themselves. They describe a research group, but we could equally well have included service users who form their own self-managed service delivery organisations. Furr gives some pointers as to what it takes to support citizens and gives some inspiring examples of what they can achieve – for themselves as well as for public services locally. Keep, with wide-ranging experience, demonstrates in different ways what it takes to bring different worlds together. Gilbert is particularly challenging in his portrayal of the involvement industry and the limited contribution that academic research has seemed to offer. Nevertheless, research is beginning to show what changes we need to make before the benefits from bringing these worlds together can be more fully demonstrated.

Creating a dialogue across difference

Back in 2002, the National Institute for Clinical Excellence (NICE) recruited '30 ordinary citizens' for a forum to consider the values that should underpin their work. Few knew anything about NICE, some were entirely unfamiliar with committee etiquette with its catching-the-eye of the chair and its turn-taking rules. A detailed study of the first meetings (Davies et al, 2006) revealed participants repeatedly puzzling about the meaning of the rather abstract topics to be discussed. They were unsure about what kinds of questions to put to the experts who gave formal presentations to them – they tried emulating TV interviewer styles – and they felt uneasy about drawing on their own experience, which seemed to be 'just anecdote'. The researchers concluded that there was a clash of different kinds of discourse and an absence of 'expertise space' to provide participants with secure grounds for making interventions. All this was despite the immense time and effort put in by the host organisations and by a facilitation team. "I don't understand what they don't understand" was the puzzled comment at one stage from the host.

Confusion can stem from different potential roles. Litva et al (2009) found that people can act as advocates, bringing their insider knowledge to bear to improve the situation for service users like themselves. People can act as consumers, gaining information to improve their own access to the best healthcare. Finally, they can act as citizens, guardians of taxpayers' money, seeking improvements for the community as a whole. This last is closest perhaps to the model of dispassionate debate and listening to evidence to which the formally organised healthcare world aspires. There are certainly positives in working with advocates. Sines illustrates this in the opening contribution to this section. But advocates can be 'passionate participants', their emotion-laden contributions can also bring an unwelcome and embarrassing disruption to routine ways of doing things. As the author of that concept argues, however, it is crucially important to acknowledge and accommodate people rather than simply rule them out of order (Barnes, 2008).

Colliding worlds place everyone outside their comfort zone. A Canadian study, for example, found health service managers struggling with how best to obtain public input through consultations (Abelson et al, 2002). These managers did not always agree among themselves on the purposes of a consultation exercise. They tended to highlight risks – the raising of expectations to an unrealistic level, for example – more than advantages. Some of the same research team went on to examine public involvement in the assessment of new health technologies. Again, they found uncertainty about appropriate ways of doing things and how to fit this into complicated constraints and accountability structures (Gauvin et al, 2010). 'Uninformed', 'too subjective' and 'unprofessional' are some of the labels that start to be used from within about those outside the provider world; 'inflexible', 'manipulative' and 'bureaucratic' come from the world outside. Dialogue requires adjustment and, as Keep points out, new language and new skills are necessary.

Asking the basic question

Litva's advocates, consumers and citizens were finding their own answers to the question: 'Why are we here?'. When it is a matter of bringing service users and citizens into the governance of a service – into the ways decisions are being made about its operation – the rewards can be several (see the following box). Too often, however, the why question is ducked or just seen as one more 'must do', with the result that everyone is in the dark.

Why involve service users and citizens in the governance of services?

- To broaden awareness of the diversity of needs in a local community.
- To prompt new ideas – including the small changes that might make a big difference in improving the experience of a service.
- To keep the focus on the fundamental purpose of the public service.
- To rehearse the reasoning for choosing a course of action and to explore unanticipated consequences.
- To promote more local understanding of dilemmas of service delivery and enhance the legitimacy of policy and service delivery decisions.

It is only when those inside an organisation have a clear sense of the value of bringing different worlds together, and are able to convey this, that they will have the motivation to enable real dialogue to occur. Tailor-made background papers, for example, can bring in newcomers in a way that conventional committee papers cannot. Issues might need to be presented through patient stories. Chairing becomes ultra-important in welcoming and acknowledging different kinds of contributions. The skills of effective facilitation (see Sims and Reed, Section 5) will at times need to be brought in from experts. Time will be required to draw out implications from the messy material that emerges from a meeting – allowing for a revisiting of issues after the outsiders have had time to reflect among themselves and perhaps to consult with stakeholders. Innovative organisational practices like this help make shared decision-making a reality. Again, the distilled key points by Keep are both relevant and practical.

Perhaps it is not surprising that local government, with its blending of bureaucratic procedures and local electoral accountability, has been quicker than the NHS to experiment with what dialogue across difference entails (Stewart, 1996). Aspects of the necessary organisational redesign can also be found in third-sector organisations and health interest groups, and in organising volunteers. But all this is rarely well-established. Learmonth et al (2009) offer a vignette from their research concerning a health authority task group reviewing local maternity services that needed an urgent meeting in view of mounting press interest. On the first proposed date, a key volunteer member was having her hair done; on the second, she had promised to look after grandchildren; on the third, she had arranged to go shopping. It is all too easy for us to see this as confirmation of the unreliability of volunteers, rather than an indicator that the organisation of the task group needed to move away from a full-time employee model.

Questions of representation and accountability

One key area where we need a new take on an old problem is in relation to representation. Well-established traditions of parliamentary democracy and local government give us the familiar idea of the elected representative as someone voted into office by members of a defined community, and who in due course can be voted out if s/he does not reflect community concerns. The 'PPI representative' is in a more ambiguous position, arriving at the table perhaps through a public appointments procedure, perhaps through getting involved in a local service group, perhaps being spotted by a service provider as someone who might have something to offer, or as being the only person in a legislatively protected category that anyone in the organisation was able to find! Unwelcome ideas from such persons can always be challenged with the question, 'How can we know that what you are saying is representative?'. A variant of this is to turn to a member of an under-represented category and ask: 'What will [women, ethnic minorities, disabled people etc] say to this?'. The response can then be met with an objection about who the speaker can be said to represent. Challenges of these sorts – consciously or not – effectively silence a participant, and often homogenise diverse communities too. It is rare that understanding of an issue is advanced.

There is another way to look at it, exemplified in recent research on faith communities (Chapman and Lowndes, 2009). A non-elected faith representative is increasingly invited to the policy table to discuss the shape of local government services, including health and social care services. What, realistically, can such a person bring? They might broaden thinking by alerting policymakers to sensitivities and to previously unconsidered reactions to policy issues by persons of faith. With good networks and personal contacts, they may be able to anticipate reactions from faith groups other than their own. They can sometimes open doors to direct contact with groups of stakeholders whom policymakers would otherwise find impossible to reach. What they cannot realistically be expected to do is speak for whole communities. This suggests that in securing the benefits of participation as set out in the box earlier, bringing in people who can tap into a variety of networks – aiming, in other words, for diversity – is altogether more appropriate than searching for the perfect representative. Malik Gul (in Section 5) offers a vivid additional example.

It is frequently said in despairing tones that an invitation to participate just produces 'the usual suspects', the few who will repeatedly turn out and whose views are not going to reflect those of the majority to be served. This, again, implies a quest for *the* representative. In practice, the usual suspects turn out to be more varied than this suggests. John May (2007) draws a triangle of engagement. At its apex are the establishment few (eg the non-executives), below them office-holders and chairs of community groups, then activists, then semi-regulars often seen at consultation events, and, finally, a much larger number who will engage if the issue is important enough.

The bottom line for public sector organisations is defensible decision-making. Yes, such organisations must routinely account for their decisions and performance 'upwards' to a government department and a minister. Increasingly, however, they must attend to accountability outwards – towards a local community. A well-constituted service-user group, with ways of reaching affected communities, can anticipate issues and help present defensible decisions in context. This will not eliminate the controversy around a hard decision, but it will demonstrate that views have been heard, add understanding of the reasoning behind the decision and, ultimately, increase trust in the inclusiveness of the governance process that has given rise to it. User co-design of specific services (see, eg, Dale in Section 2 and Gul in Section 5) takes this thinking further.

Guidelines and toolkits now abound (as Gilbert points out in this section). Their hints about the pros and cons of different techniques of engagement are helpful. But they are no substitute for recognition of what it takes for colliding worlds to engage, hard thinking about objectives in a specific context and a welcome for the multiplicity, inherent 'messiness' and slow relationship-building that produces novel insights and ideas.

Collaborative governance – coming into sight?

The colliding-world encounters that are the present experience of so much that goes under the heading of public engagement are not taking place in a vacuum. The terrains of local government, local voluntary action and the NHS are increasingly overlapping through the creation of partnerships for area regeneration and the arrival of new players in the service delivery mix. Writing in 2008, Barnes and her colleagues estimated that there were in the region of 75,000 partnership board places in the UK where input from local residents and local users of services was being required. They pointed out that the training of public service managers had not caught up (Barnes et al, 2008, p 71).

Research is putting a name to this, in the shape of citizen-centred, inclusive or participatory or collaborative governance. Collaborative governance, according to a US study pulling more than 130 examples together from across many sectors, is an arrangement:'[W]here one or more public agencies directly engage non-state stakeholders in a collective decision-making process that is formal, consensus-oriented, and deliberative, and that aims to make or implement public policy or manage public programs or assets' (Ansell and Gash, 2008, p 544).

Today's complexity of powers, responsibilities and accountabilities has gone beyond the bureaucratic hierarchies and professional autonomy of the health service or formal chains of political accountability through periodic elections of local government. Our organisational arrangements and skill sets, however, are at the very beginning of reflecting this.

Supporters of PPI, as noted at the outset, have moved to use of the term 'engagement' to replace involvement, in recognition of how often involvement ends up as a sham. The newer term has its own ambiguities, however. Neither military engagement (with the other as enemy) nor marital engagement (with the other as hoped-for perfect consort) hits the right spot. Motor engagement (the meshing of gears of different sizes enabling the vehicle to go faster) is perhaps the best metaphor of the three. New words need to be accompanied by the new practices or actions that they signal.

At the time of writing this piece (winter 2011/12), another reorganisation of governance arrangements for PPI was under way. Much time and effort will be expended over the coming years putting into place Health and Wellbeing Boards, establishing how they will work with Overview and Scrutiny arrangements, where local Healthwatch will fit in, what arrangements there will be at national level and so on. Building collaborative governance within these structures can be done. The onus is on those working within the health and social care services to think strategically, to step into the worlds of those with whom they need to work and build the skills and support (for themselves as well as for others) to ensure real engagement between professional practice and the everyday.

SECTION 4

How can information technology work for well-being? Data, dialogues and digital media

Introduction

No area within healthcare is more riven with 'compulsory innovation' than information and communications technologies (ICTs). The field impinges on all healthcare fields and sectors, since any medical service involves some kind of 'information service' where ICTs might figure: a hospital discharge letter, a database of lab results, some performance statistics or even an old-fashioned conversation between doctor and patient or between colleagues.

This section is assembled around the notion that healthcare innovation that is beneficial to well-being (as distinct from the endless churn of compulsory innovation) results from engagement of service users and their advocates in ensuring and delivering quality, and, especially, from engagement that takes the form of self-management. Dialogue is central. In this section, we explore some ways in which digital data and digital media enable and shape engagement in dialogues around quality; also, some ways in which engagement in and commitment to dialogues underlies the creation of new ICT systems. The chapters fall into two sets. The first set focuses on systems that handle private information about specific patients and their treatments; the second is concerned with how ICTs are being used to handle public information, commentary and assessments of performance.

The first two chapters focus on medical records in the GP sector. **Yvonne Bennett** writes as a patient, highlighting how online access to electronic patient records (EPRs) can directly contribute to well-being by helping people to make sense of things in their personal and family life. **Brian Fisher** is also enthusiastic about the potential of access to EPRs but he underlines how clinicians tend to feel challenged by the shifts of status and privilege that are involved, and sees this as an obstacle to benefit for patients. Finally in this first set, **Lawrence Goldberg** discusses how clinicians and others in the hospital sector have managed to generate and sustain dialogue across organisational boundaries, developing a system of electronic patient records in kidney care, integrated at the regional level. He highlights an endemic difficulty in finding relevant facilitation skills within the NHS, and notes that there is a road yet to be travelled to meet expectations of patient and carer involvement in developing ICT tools. Developments are uneven. Writing from the primary care sector, Fisher is optimistic about timescales for patients' access to digital records; Goldberg's view from the hospital sector is more cautious.

The remaining chapters explore how stories about the NHS appear in the public domain via digital media, or get woven around published data and accounts. **Tris Taylor** notes how mobile phone 'apps' are increasingly able to find, mine and assemble data of many different kinds across the Internet (official statistics, users' comments and tags, digital images, geographically based compilations of documents and data). He states a challenge that medical professionals will need to respond to as they increasingly encounter patients who carry these toolkits around in their pockets and handbags. **Neil Bacon** develops a related argument about the expectations of people who approach medical care in the same spirit that they make choices in the marketplace, regarding the quality of the hotel or car they want to use. In contrast, **Paul Hodgkin** explores how a 'storytelling' service based on digital media can embody a different kind of economics: gift-giving. Finally, after three chapters that embrace the capacity of ICTs to pull and push digital documents across the Internet, **Valerie Iles** takes a step back. Picking up on the same trends in cheapness, capacity, data-crunching and digital distribution as the previous three contributors, she argues that these can result in a kind of dumbing down that helps undermine the exercise of thoughtful, purposeful judgement.

Closing the section, editor **Mike Hales** highlights challenges to professional and organisational culture in healthcare arising from ICT-based innovations. He suggests that with regard to leadership, orienting to cultural as distinct from technological innovations is central.

23

Records help us make sense of our lives

Yvonne Bennett

There is a change in the National Health Service that you either embrace or loathe. Today's patient is more than ever not only wanting but demanding to be at the centre of their own healthcare. Patients want to be treated not as an arm or a leg, but as a whole person. They want to take part in a true consultation where both partners are equal with a different quality of expertise.

Access to health records has opened up a larger insight for the patient. Years ago, at the age of 31, one patient was assured that they must have been in a road accident as their spine was flat instead of curved. The patient was adamant that they hadn't. Thirty-odd years later, in their sixties, they were allowed access to their medical records – and the mystery was solved: an entry in their records for a greenstick fracture of the left arm as a child. At this prompt, the patient remembered that they had fallen from a tree. Although the fracture was the only thing recorded, they did remember that they spent a long time off school. They were extremely sore for weeks and for a while had difficulty walking. The 'road accident' spine was explained.

Patients may be seen at different hospitals or by different consultants at the same hospital. It's the patient who can supply all the information as they are there from beginning to end. When a person is attending a consultation for a foot complaint, there are very often other factors that fit into the equation. In general, patients are happy to share their information with clinicians so it is important that patients have access to their medical records. It is beneficial not only to patients, but to clinicians too, and it is cost-effective and time-saving for both: no need to repeat tests unnecessarily or take up extra appointments.

I attended the fracture clinic at my local hospital because I had broken my shoulder. I had previously broken the same shoulder and was treated at a different hospital. When I was seen by the osteoporosis specialist nurse, I was able to take my previous dexa scan (done at a different hospital, and not available to the nurse). She found this fascinating and practical, so much so that she phoned someone at the Primary Care Trust to tell them how good this was. The nurse was able to decide whether a repeat scan was needed, or whether advice and treatment could start immediately. I was also able to give the physiotherapist a report from the previous hospital detailing the range of movement achieved after the previous fracture.

Family history plays an important role in healthcare. Many have 'long-term conditions' but a strong family history of diabetes, heart disease or strokes may have more significance for a patient and form part of their picture of health and well-being. It is good for parents to hand on to their children information about family health. As medicine is constantly improving, genetic information may prove to be a life-saving factor for a future generation. I have a 12-year-old grandson and our family history may be important to him in later life.

With access to the Internet, patients, young or old, are now understanding their own health and that of their loved ones. A person who discovers a 'mysterious lump' is more likely to ask a relative or friend, or try the Internet, before they get round to the GP. This isn't because they don't trust the GP, but more likely because they aren't sure of themselves, and don't want to waste time. Easy access to medical records is all part of the picture that helps us make sense of our lives – in the years gone by and in the present day, with the GP and at the hospital, inheriting things and passing things on within our families, exploring things with friends.

There are many champions out there, be they medical workers or just members of the public, who want a top-quality service. Long may they all continue.

24

Records access and empowered patients, 2017

Brian Fisher

Your personal health record makes your healthcare more efficient and safe – a dream? Here is a vision:

> 2017: we are five years in the future. People have routine access to their own health records from primary and secondary healthcare. They can store and share them, comment on them, add their own data.
>
> People use this access to save time, gain knowledge, get support in looking after their own health, plan their care, communicate with their clinicians and improve the accuracy and relevance of the data. They share their record with selected others to ensure integrated care and information where it is needed.
>
> The health record becomes a personalised portal to a wide range of online software applications that can interact with your record and generate guidance based on your own self-monitored data: blood pressure, peak flow, weight and so on.
>
> The record becomes a route through which the NHS can communicate personally with you, sending you messages that help you improve your health and offering you opportunities to use services in or out of the NHS. You can see which practices offer access. You can use the record to find out more about the quality of the practices in your area.
>
> Clinicians throughout the NHS harness record access to offer safer, more efficient care. From their point of view, empowered patients are easier 'cases' to manage, achieve better outcomes and use NHS services less.

Much of this is possible now

We are only a few steps away from this vision. Right now, it is possible for 60% of GP practices in the UK to give patients access to their full record online for free; it is part of the patient-information system (EMIS) that they already subscribe to. Even though it contains everything your GP holds about you electronically, your patient's display of the record is reformatted in ways that patients have explained are most easy to understand.

It is essential that people not only have access to data, but also are able to understand it and make use of it. If you understand what a myocardial infarction is, you can do much more about it than if you don't. In the PAERS/EMIS system, every Read code is linked to patient information leaflets as well as relevant national patient organisations. You don't have to trawl the net; relevant, accredited information is at your fingertips – a personalised, automated information prescription. 'Information buttons' in the record click through to sources of further information. The same applies to test results (eg cholesterol tests) viewed through the system.

In this system you can copy and share. You can correct the data by contacting your practice. You can ensure that the data is available to those people who need it – your clinicians, your carers, your family.

There are other examples of record access in the UK:

- *Patients Know Best*. Available at: www.patientsknowbest.com
- *Renal Patient View*, where UK renal departments can offer patients access to aspects of their hospital record. Available at: www.renalpatientview.org
- *HealthSpace*, where the NHS portal will enable patients to see their Summary Care Record. Available at: www.healthspace.nhs.uk/visitor

Clinicians are challenged by this

This is a real information revolution, and a challenge for clinicians. Most of the experience in the UK has been with GPs, whose first reaction to a discussion on records access is anxiety. GPs have a range of concerns.

The first worry is that records access will result in extra work. GPs fear that patients will need more and longer appointments to discuss trivial aspects of the record. Evidence suggests that this does not generally happen. Experience in the UK and theUS is similar.

The second worry is that records access will result in more litigation. The concern is that patients will more easily pick up mistakes and red herrings and will sue. In fact, it seems that litigation rates do not increase.

The third worry is that patients will see third-party information that they should not see under the Data Protection Act. The reality is that there are technical arrangements and small changes in administration that reduce the risk to almost zero.

GPs' fourth worry is more deep-seated: this is such a profound shift in the balance of forces that we should proceed, if at all, with great caution. Who knows what might happen if we forgo our privileged access to this personal information? In fact, clinicians who have taken the steps into access find it a liberating and straightforward experience. It enables easier, safer, better practice.

Patients like it

Patients, on the other hand, have an almost universally good experience of records access. There is evidence of pleasure, efficiencies, improved safety, improved self-care and a feeling of being more in control of their lives and their healthcare.

Improved self-care

Clinicians and patients agree that patients look after themselves better with records access. There is evidence of greater success at giving up smoking and continuing to take medication. Anecdotally, people say that seeing the clinician's advice in black and white on their notes, particularly when linked with supporting information that aids understanding, makes a big difference to behaving differently.

Safer care

Patients correct their records (though it would be better if this happened more). They share the record in accident and emergency settings in the UK and abroad. They share with out-patient departments, gluing different parts of the NHS together. Care homes can enable visiting out-of-hours clinicians to have access to the key data when they visit in the night. No longer do night visits have to be 'in the dark' with information.

Shared decision-making

People are better informed, better motivated and can use the record in an intelligent way to get the best out of NHS in a positive and engaged way.

Saving time

No telephoning for results, no need to check whether a referral has been made, no calling for the consultant's letter – it's all there. Combined with the ability to book appointments and repeat prescriptions, this begins to approach a service fit for the 21st century. It saves time for patients, and there is some evidence that it saves time for practices too. Fewer telephone calls is an obvious saving. In the US, there is evidence that combining records access and secure messaging substantially reduces telephone calls and appointments.

Government policy

Records access has been government policy since 2000. The current government has emphasised access as a key theme. In addition, they emphasise 'control' over the patient's record. By this, they perhaps mean the patient's ability to copy and share; to be able to share different parts of their record with different people; and to hold both clinician initiated-data such as your GP record and data you have collected yourself, such as your home blood pressure. Sadly, HealthSpace (part of NHS Connecting for Health) appears effectively to have failed. It will offer patients access to the thinnest of data and the evidence is that this is insufficient to be useful to patients. However, the Treasury may still fund it.

The future

We are on the verge of a new world: a Web 2.0 interactive record. It will soon be possible for patients to add securely to their electronic patient record. Organisations such as GP consortia and GP practices will be able to send health promotion messages to their patients that will be tailored to their needs. For instance, messages about stopping smoking will be seen only by smokers – automated social marketing. Third parties will be able to create gadgets that automatically and securely use key data from the record to help you look after yourself better in a personalised and effective manner.

How can we help advance this information revolution? We are only in the foothills of making this kind of approach as useful as it can be to professionals and patients. The main limiter is resistance from the medical profession. One approach is to work closely with clinicians to overcome preconceptions and make switching as easy as possible. The Health Foundation is funding a Closing the Gap project in Lewisham to look in detail at how best to shift the dynamic between clinicians and their patients with respect to patients' information.

The NHS is considering a national programme to raise the profile of records access, encouraging not only a 'push' for clinicians but also a 'pull' from patients:

- *Patients*: contact your GP now – ask for records access. If their practice cannot offer it now, ask them to contact their IT supplier to make it possible. If you are in the 60% of UK practices who can offer it now, urge and cajole them.
- *Health organisations*: this is one of the simplest, most effective ways of encouraging self-care and shared decision-making. Urge and support your practices to offer records access now.
- *GP practices*: be reassured. This is a simple, safe and effective approach to offering better care to your patients and obtaining the benefits of informed and involved patients. Offer records access if you can.

We shall see an empowered active population who can use their record as a way of taking more control over their NHS, sharing control of data about themselves and sharing benefits with the professionals.

25

Learning to build a high-quality information system to support high-quality renal care

Lawrence Goldberg

In the care of long-term medical conditions, we need to deliver ever-higher-quality and safer care, as efficiently as possible, in a way that gives patients the opportunity to be informed and involved in the management of their own conditions. Proactive disease management – in which deteriorations in health parameters are detected early and intervention is prompt – is all-important to avoid acute and severe illness developing. Quality, safety and efficiency in healthcare are all aligned.

This chapter summarises some experience and learning within a hospital-based specialty about how to deliver these goals. Over the last six years or so, we have worked to develop information systems to support the care of patients with kidney disease in Sussex, from a regional hospital specialty perspective. In the following, we consider three areas of learning:

- Discovering how people from different spheres can work together and innovate (through action learning).
- Being pragmatic in scoping and integrating the electronic patient record.
- Getting together to define what quality looks like in the future (through skilled facilitation and user engagement).

Action learning

Following the publication of a National Service Framework, we won Department of Health funding to set up an action learning set to work on a long-term care pathway for chronic kidney disease, drawing in members from primary and secondary care. Getting stakeholders together in this way was unfamiliar then, and is still somewhat counter-cultural within the NHS, with its hierarchies and boundaries. It can be hard to get authorised time in the working week for action learning. External backing – and funding – meant that the Trust's Chief Executive was much more willing to give the go-ahead for an experiment in working together in a new way.

Action learning sets are an excellent context for blue-skies thinking; an explicit and protected opportunity to think freely and discuss new ways of working with people you otherwise would see only in formal meetings with formal agendas. They provide a collaborative environment in which to help meet individuals' and the group's challenges, generate and test new ideas, assess the feasibility of doing things that previously seemed impossible, and discover who to talk to.

Our learning set brought seven or eight busy people from different settings together in a regular diary slot: a consultant and business manager from the hospital, a patient, and, from primary care, a GP, a Primary Care Trust (PCT) lead, a practice nurse and a commissioner. The set was inspirationally facilitated by Bob Sang, who ensured that the patients' perspective, and ideas around patient self-management, remained in the fore.

Previously, managing kidney disease had been mainly a specialist area that GPs had left to hospitals. In fact, much of the care can be undertaken within primary care without the need for face-to-face specialists' involvement. The learning set aimed to simplify the care pathways and develop educational tools to enable GPs to undertake the long-term care of kidney patients, especially when their condition is stable. This work anticipated some of the new quality targets that were coming out for GPs and ensured that the local primary care sector was ahead of the game when the national GP targets came along.

Practice nurses are key to managing chronic disease: they run the annual reviews, and they are the first point of contact for many patients with chronic conditions. A key understanding, which emerged particularly from practice nurses' ways of working, was the need in the hospital sector to integrate care across specialist 'silos'. Many patients have more than one chronic disease, with a lot of overlap in clinical management. It is not uncommon for a patient to have heart disease, diabetes and chronic kidney disease, and for all three, best care involves good blood pressure and cholesterol control, lifestyle advice about smoking, weight reduction, and exercise. There are clear benefits from integrating these fundamental aspects of care. Patients benefit further from minimising visits to different clinics. This learning influenced Department of Health thinking, and the formation by the 'Tsars' (National Clinical Directors) of heart disease, diabetes, stroke and renal medicine of a national Vascular Board.

More recently, we created another action learning set to progress the goals of the Sussex Renal Innovation Programme, which is implementing modernised practices in the day-to-day operations of our unit. While there is a formal project board, the learning set is the engine of innovation. It meets monthly and comprises a multidisciplinary group of healthcare professionals within the hospital, together with patients and a representative of the health informatics department (given the key enabling role of information technology [IT]).

Once again, the renal department gained a degree of autonomy to organise in this way, through support (seedcorn money) provided by the Strategic Health Authority and the local PCT. This autonomy insulated us somewhat from the bureaucracy that always holds a risk of killing innovation, vision and flexibility (eg we've kept alongside, but not been dominated by, the IT department). Availability of time continues to be an issue. Some clinicians participate in their free time because of the value they attach to the dialogue. We don't have the means to pay patients for their time, but we acknowledge it with department store vouchers and travel expenses; visibly valuing patients' time has been a principle of the project. Nursing staff make time available through scheduling and the support of their line managers.

Electronic patient records – crossing boundaries

There is now international recognition of the potential to dramatically enhance the quality, safety and efficiency of healthcare delivery and management by storing and accessing data and documents in electronic form. Healthcare is delivered in many settings by many people, each using their own systems, usually paper-based. Information about patients and their current condition is often in the wrong place at the wrong time, and not always consistent, which generates risks. Everything is interconnected in patient care – the social side, medical, financial – and if information is all there, it is so much easier for those caring for patients to 'manage the whole patient' rather than working in the silo of a single disease approach. Relevant clinical and other information can be connected up and made available across multiple sites in real time by storing data and documentation electronically in an electronic patient record (EPR).

The Holy Grail is a single comprehensive and instantly analysable patients' database, accessible to all involved in the care of individual patients – including patients. The NHS is a long way from achieving this. GP surgeries have had electronic systems for some time but they do not relate to each other or to their health and social care partners. Hospitals are at last looking to introduce EPRs but do not look as though they will be able to integrate with other systems in the community. There is duplicated information, inconsistency, an inherent risk of error and inefficiency.

The renal unit, along with other tertiary specialties, is responsible for patients referred across a wide geographical area spanning East and West Sussex. Patients attend their GP surgery and local hospital, not just the specialists in Brighton. In this situation, data from lab tests can be fragmented in a very unhelpful way. Laboratory results – blood tests, for example – are often a vital component of the information needed to manage long-term conditions and underpin dialogues between specialists, GPs and patients. The current fragmented storage of this data compromises coordinated, preventative care, and introduces risks of error and duplication. We have focused on pulling in laboratory data from the hospitals in our region to a single database, and have brought together representatives of clinicians, laboratory staff from the three hospitals, the commercial EPR software provider and the IT department. Once established, the benefits of this laboratory integration will be widely shared well beyond the renal service.

The ability to fully analyse the EPR in a whole range of ways is critical to maximise the benefits. This is a point often missed by those who design systems, who are not involved with the day-to-day use of data in managing a patient's illness. It is so important to be able to look at trends, what's happening over time, how they've responded to a particular treatment, in relation to clinical parameters (their diabetes, their anaemia), the drugs they're on, infections they might have had. Are they stable or deteriorating? Tools to pick up things early (pre-clinically, prior to the patient developing symptoms) can enable quick intervention, safer treatment, higher quality and cost-effective care. It can also directly enable better quality of life for the patient – for example, by avoiding an admission to hospital, enabling them to stay at home or enabling them to stay at work.

Although the ambition for a comprehensive EPR is clear, a Big Bang approach is doomed to fail. The National Programme for IT foundered on this overambition. Our approach has been a local and staged development. The key has been to start with getting an EPR to work highly effectively within a single clinical area (in our case, kidney disease) but, also vitally, shared with patients. The next tier of ambition then looks to spread access to other specialties responsible for long-term conditions that tend to occur together, such as diabetes, cardiology and cancer, to enable 'patient-centric care'. The third and most challenging tier of ambition is to look at how to integrate and harmonise with clinical information systems external to the hospital: GP, community and social care. Even the big commercial health informatics players, who are implementing EPR systems in the NHS, are putting them in as hospital-based systems, not integrating across into primary care and the community. There are huge challenges arising from different coding systems and ways of defining and recording health events and outcomes.

There needs to be a degree of realism, pragmatism, flexibility and localism in approach, as distinct from ploughing ahead with top-down visions and specifications, formulated – and to some extent 'hardened' – on a national level and pitched at all three tiers of integrated EPR development. Although in this section Brian Fisher writes optimistically about the timescale for patients' access to their EPR in the primary care sector, integration across sectors seems to be running on a longer timescale. Primary care has been waiting for secondary care to 'catch up' with their progress, to the point where there is good-quality, relevant digital data about patients' conditions and treatments that might be meaningfully shared.

Throughout our work in this area, the key has been to ensure that users remain pivotal and influential in developing and specifying the clinical system that they will be using. In developing a user-led specification, we've consulted with GPs, other specialists and patients. We've also been aware of the value of getting something in and working, within a hospital, within an individual specialty, and then broadening out this working base of technology and practice, in an evolutionary way, through expanded dialogues around a working model. It's partly a question of confidence-building: you can promote ideas or a vision out into the community or across a hospital and people will just walk the other way because there's such a history of failed health informatics projects, disappointed expectations and oversold technology. When there's a working version of technology and practice, it's much easier for potential users in adjacent domains to see what it is that will actually be useful for them in an extended system.

For example, the response of GPs locally often can be: 'We've had digital records for years, it's familiar, there's no need for anything different.' But systems in the primary care sector don't reach across the primary–secondary care division. Our experience has been that it may take a working demonstration of a system that can potentially talk across that gap before they 'get' the issue and feel that it makes sense to engage in a conversation about change and expanded ambitions.

Quality, participation and facilitation in the future

Throughout, we have recognised that quality – of information systems, of clinical information, of care – arises from (often novel, sometimes difficult) dialogues between stakeholders across primary and secondary care and in the community. We've learned a great deal in going down our route to achieve the solution we currently have, which is still somewhat limited in scope and function (eg operating only among staff within a single specialty, limited capacity for real-time analysis). Even with this experience, though, there are questions about where the capacity resides to establish and expand the dialogues that will be needed to create the system we ultimately need – operating at the third tier, across primary and secondary care and in the community, fully supporting cost-reducing, proactive disease management using sophisticated analysis of timelines, and supporting the practice of NHS staff and patients alike through appropriate means of access.

Getting together to define what quality looks like remains challenging (Section Two has more to say on this). There continues to be a lot of top-down defining of quality by the NHS, with localities reporting back up within the hierarchy. As GP commissioning (now *clinical commissioning*) takes off, and we develop much more clinician-to-clinician partnership working, then involving patients in that is going to be critical.

We now understand that facilitation of dialogue or the design and execution of group processes are in themselves skills outside of the usual clinical professional field, lying beyond the kinds of professional competencies typically found in the NHS. More people in this organisation are familiar now with the kinds of strategies and techniques that can be used to conduct dialogues among stakeholders, but many clinicians and managers still find this foreign and 'soft'. The willingness to trust and engage in processes of learning and exploration across usual boundaries, which may be quite well known in 'the outside world' (like action learning), is not yet deeply embedded in our own culture. In furthering our project's aims for quality and integration, and the dialogues they depend on, I am not sure that we yet know where to look for these essential skills.

For us, after six years of learning, it has now become much more instinctive to get people talking and sharing ideas outside a formal machinery of meetings, agendas and performance measures for 'participation'. Patient and public involvement – 'PPI' – is ubiquitous. But dealing with this through the formal structures and roles of institutional machinery does not necessarily deliver the kind of engagement, or finely textured working relationships between people, that we have learned to value in building a high-quality information system to support high-quality renal care.

26

Embracing social technology

Tris Taylor

Before long, I will be able to get off the bus at the hospital, turn on my phone and, as I walk through the doors, flick through ratings and comments by carers, patients, staff and the press. When I check in at reception, I'll be able to hold my phone up to the receptionist and have a little display of how he or she is characterised by others who have been here. Before I set off, I'll have read up on whether or not the people I am here to see are punctual, and if they're not, I may have chosen to arrive later than my appointed time.

When I get into the consulting room, I'll be able to see on my phone some of the people who have been here before me, glance at the headlines of the opinions they have expressed about their experiences, and check that the consultant sitting in front of me is the one they are talking about. If I judge from what I see and read that I am in good hands, I'll sit down ready to talk. If not, I'll steel myself for a bit of a wrestle, and if I have to walk out, I'll feel better about doing so.

This is how it's going to be. The technologies exist now: face recognition, geographical tagging and location check-ins, official ratings data and customer ratings sites, clever programs that access lots of different data sources and present you with an easily digestible analysis, and mobile phones that can handle this stuff easily. Very soon, probably before this book is published, someone is going to write an app or develop a website that brings all this and more to my fingertips; and that will open the gates for lots of other companies to make even better ones.

My tip to you if you work in health is to go along with it. You have an absolute right to privacy in your personal life. At work, it is different. If you are going to be involved in decisions about my health, it is reasonable and responsible to expect that I should be able to access information about your working practices and results as part of my making a judgement about entering into a working relationship with you. If you try to avoid making information available, I will find that suspicious.

So, use social websites to link yourself (in the virtual world) to your educational establishments and places of work, your special interests, your professional successes and failures, your publications and professional opinions. Keep private your social life, hobbies and family – they are none of my business. And continue to maintain the confidentiality of our relationship – but be prepared for the eventuality that I choose to make that link public.

Be honest and fear not. I am looking for things I can believe, respect and understand. I am not always going to be in a good mood, but then neither are you. We are humans trying to relate to one another in a professional context, and some of this technology is going to make things easier.

Over to you!

27

Enlightening the next user

Neil Bacon

Buying a house or car, booking a holiday or hotel ... social changes and the power of the Internet have created an informed public whose members make choices and demand transparent information on which to base them. A key part of that information is the shared opinion and experience of others. If your restaurant is dirty or your airline staff are rude, your customer may share their experience on a public website for millions to see at the click of a Google search. Get things right, go the extra mile, deliver excellence – then the same customer will likely record this positive view.

In just a couple of years such behaviour – and the value it brings to both the public and providers – has become totally accepted across nearly all industries. How many of us would even consider staying in a hotel that refused to be rated by its clients, or buy from an eBay seller who somehow blocked anyone from giving them a rating and feedback? Citizen power has transformed services across sectors, driving quality up and costs down, giving providers instant, detailed understanding of the perceptions of their users, and ensuring the best thrive and the worst improve or go bust. It is hard to think of a single industry where robust, systematic user feedback, shared fully across the Internet, has not driven an improvement in its services. Health and social care stands in isolation as the only significant sector where such opportunities have yet to be realised. Making clinical outcome information available to the public is increasingly recognised as an important first step in helping our citizens understand the variation in quality that exists across the NHS.

Like any large organisation, there will always be a spread of performance. A small number of doctors or hospitals are excellent, a small number awful; most are somewhere between, delivering distinctly average care. The important thing is to be able to recognise this variation, reduce it and improve the outcomes at every level. But how can the public properly understand what sort of care their local GP, dentist or hospital provides, let alone be part of a process of improving the quality?

Some would say that sort of improvement programme should be left to the government, hospitals and medical professions. However, evidence suggests otherwise. Perhaps in this case, rather than the doctor, it is the patient who knows best.

In order to start this information revolution, citizens need unfettered access to two sorts of information: clinical outcome and performance data (hospital infection rates, cancer survival figures, etc) and the shared experiences of other patients. The Department of Health's own efforts in this respect (through the Care Quality Commission, its predecessors and NHS Choices) highlight the extent of big government's ineffectiveness in such areas. Central provision of so-called comparative information to support patient choice has been shown by the government's own figures to be expensive and ineffectual in empowering the public and improving quality. At best, they have been confusing and, at worst, misleading, with hospitals passed by inspectors with good scores subsequently being shown to be dangerous and poorly run.

More work needs to be done to define the top three or four clinical outcomes that multidisciplinary healthcare teams – and their patients – would deem the most important for conditions like asthma, diabetes and cancer, in terms of returning maximum health gain. But we have access to some of the best clinical teams on the planet, who we should exercise to generate these outcomes.

Sharing data on clinical outcomes alone – an important and necessary step – will not be sufficient. How can people make intelligent choices for themselves and their families? Radical knowledge-based transformation of the NHS has already started in a few areas of the UK and may be about to expand and spread like other Internet phenomena such as Twitter or MySpace. In Wales, all those using the palliative care and hospice services (patients and carers) provide continuous feedback on their care using an online service. After a year-long pilot, it has been extended to include data collection online and offline, in both English and Welsh. In the 2010 'information revolution' consultation paper (Department of Health 2010d), the Department of Health outlined how harnessing the power of patients could create the change that top-down targets have failed to do, and he cited iWantGreatCare.org (iWantGreatCare, 2011) as an example of the sort of innovative approach needed to deliver the change. It's a service that makes it as easy to rate and review doctors, hospitals, dentists, pharmacists and nursing homes as it is to rate a book from Amazon or a seller on eBay.

There is nothing to stop healthcare in the UK seeing the same radical improvement and change that TripAdvisor has delivered for hotels across the world, and for the people staying in them. This will not cost a fortune; rather, it requires government to legislate that providers of care must have robust, effective, open systems to collect and share feedback on key items – not just the piecemeal, ineffective surveys that have been the norm.

It is then up to patients, their families and the associations who represent them to ask questions, demand transparency of information about effectiveness and outcomes of the care provided, and read independent opinion and ratings from other patients. The public needs to make considered choices based on this information – and then to take two minutes to give feedback, reviews and ratings on the care provided.

Enlightening the next user in this way works across other industries and will deliver a profound change in healthcare, supporting the concept of an empowered public to finally create the market needed to drive mediocrity out of the NHS.

28

Patients' stories – digital gifts that can change the world

Paul Hodgkin

When Jenny's 86-year-old mother was admitted to hospital, lunch was always sandwiches – perhaps understandable in a recession. The problem was that they came wrapped in so many layers of cling film that Jenny's mum, with her arthritic hands, couldn't get at them and so went hungry.

Jenny complained but it did not seem to make any difference to the cling film, or to her mum. In the old days, that would have been that: one more old lady leaving the NHS, grateful for the core service, less well than she might have been. But nowadays, the Internet gives people different kinds of voice, and Jenny chose to share her mum's story on the Patient Opinion website (www.patientopinion.org. uk). These mechanisms are new – what are the effects likely to be?

Back in the old days of the 20th century, Jenny would have found it expensive to have a public voice. Getting a letter published in a newspaper was the best that most of us could hope for. Today, the cost of having a public voice is zero for anyone with access to the net. There is a publishing Klondike into which have poured YouTube, FaceBook, MySpace. Economics being what it is, of course, a decrease in price of voice implies an increase in supply, which in turn creates a crowded marketplace – and all too soon people must shout to be heard. So, cheap voice alone leads not only to communication and creativity, but also to cantankerousness, insults and bullying. In economic terms, cheap voice is both a good thing (more people are involved) and a problem (the cost of hearing the real message in all the noise rises rapidly). The overall result is that in the public realm, universal voice has been much less transformative than was predicted.

For Jenny's new power of public voice to start to change the world, her story needs to get to just the right person – in this case, the catering manager – whose job it is to say 'Easy on the cling film'. Patient Opinion does this by directing stories to 'just the right person' via a flexible email alert service to the care-giving organisation. That way, busy managers can hear the signal without the noise, and sometimes patients and families get to change some significant part of the world.

From the manager's or politician's perspective, this selective listening makes a cacophony of voices much more meaningful. In economic terms, cheap voice plus highly cost-effective listening radically lower the costs of being responsive. Problems that previously were too expensive to discover or deal with have become economic no-brainers – of course, we should hold the cling film.

Not just the costs of voice – costs of collaboration too

The new economics of the web is not just about cheap voice. For citizens, the cost of collaboration is also approaching zero. As Clay Shirky says in *Here comes everybody* (Shirky, 2008), the Internet has made forming groups ridiculously easy. With cheap collaboration, groups arise that neither the market nor the previous social glue of communities could have sustained. So, people dying from advanced renal carcinoma can find each other and, in the space of eight weeks, get NICE to reverse its ban on the latest drugs.

Partly, this is due to the ease and cheapness of finding those with a common interest, partly to the ease with which cheap voice and some political nous can be allied to good effect. Overall the economics of cheap collaboration work strongly to the advantage of citizens who have the freedom and now the Internet-based tools to self-organise.

For organisations, however, the costs of collaboration are rising – witness the amount of time spent in meetings or the progressive decline in the time that health professionals spend face to face with patients. While loose coalitions of citizens are able to 'just do it', organisations are constrained by formal governance and accountability, order and history. The demand for joined-up government adds further burdens. Each additional organisation involved in delivering a policy, or each additional target, means a non-linear rise in the number of possible side effects, partners and issues to be handled.

These two trends together mean that the NHS underperforms against the possible: a dance of gnats and elephants, as ephemeral single issue groups vie to seize the media megaphone while bureaucracies lumber on, twitching irritably, changing direction occasionally. For big pubic bureaucracies like the NHS, a new swarm of motivated citizen groups, built around cheap collaboration and accessing cheap voice, sounds like a mixed blessing. Single issue monomaniacs who understand neither the subtleties nor the constraints of managing public resources could do more harm than good, and the solidarity on which the NHS is based could be undermined as each group uses its new power in an ultimately self-defeating shouting match of each against all.

Giving is fundamental

At least part of the answer lies in digital gift economies – another aspect of the new economics being midwifed by the web. Digital gift economies (like Wikipedia and Linux) are important because they manage, as if by magic, to conjure massive commitment to common ends from a small minority who willingly contribute to the good of all for no financial reward whatsoever. They have appeared because the web has lowered transaction costs by several orders of magnitude. What was once expensive (Britannica) is now free and better (Wikipedia).

Accustomed to the self-serving rhetoric of the market, we may easily feel that it's absurd that a significant part of the human world is governed by giving, not getting. In reality, gift economies lie at the heart of families, teams, friendship – in fact, much of what we value most. They are usually destroyed by money (try paying your mother-in-law for the meal she has just cooked for you). This means that they are largely invisible to markets, businesses and economists.

Giving, and the web of mutual obligation and pleasure that it creates, has provided glue within kinship groups and tribes throughout pre-history. Our predilection for giving is probably rooted in the cooperative child-rearing practices that were needed to enable hunter-gatherers to find the 13 million calories required to raise a human infant to the age of 18 in pre-agricultural societies – it's more than a couple can collect (Blaffer Hrdy, 2009). This chimes with evidence that the act of giving itself increases well-being – for example, consciously giving something away each day improves depression even if done without anyone else knowing.

Of course, people give stuff for reasons – to enhance their reputations, to create a sense of obligation. So, gift economies are run by ordinary people, not angels; but, on the other hand, they are very different from markets because the value of the gift is determined by relationship not scarcity – a handmade cake from a grandchild carries more value than the most expensive one in the shop.

Digital gift economies gain scale

Traditional gift economies don't scale well precisely because they have to be rooted in a relationship – giving stuff to strangers is a mug's game. More importantly, economies based on giving physical things tend to run out of either stuff (the empty cooking pot) or meaning (too many pairs of socks at Christmas). Till now, these constraints have limited gift economies to groups that give physical stuff within existing webs of relationships. The digital world changes this because the exchange of digital goods can access an infinite supply of free gifts. In economic terms, digital items in a gift economy are *non-rivalrous*. They are somewhat like songs – freely available and hence non-rivalrous, but usually attributed to someone (unlike classical non-rivalrous goods, which are generic, without personal attribution).

The most important effect of the web is to solve the free-rider problem. Having 250 people turn up to eat your free (physical) lunch when you were only expecting the 25 who came with food is a supply problem and an incentive nightmare. Having 25,000 people download your (digital) software rather than the 25 you wrote it for is the definition of success. In a digital world, free-riders become the audience and moral hazard becomes reputational payback.

This has profound implications for solving human problems, and understanding digital gift economies matters a lot. Partly, this is because they can be subverted: for the jihadist, suicide is the ultimate gift, dead bodies the currency and video statements the means to gain reputation. More importantly, digital gift economies are a way to *release large quantities of free resources in ways that draw us together*.

Constructing working digital gift economies is a hit-and-miss affair right now, but no matter. The point is that we are on the way home, and have found the other half of the market, the half that existed around the campfire before the market was dreamed of. Digital gift economies release creativity, action and meaning from their tribal roots and allow them to embrace the global.

Close to the heart of the NHS

Jenny probably had many reasons to send her story of the cling film to Patient Opinion. The task of dealing with it can also be seen from many perspectives – as an ethical imperative, an efficient short cut to better services, a necessary requirement of the market. But viewed as a gift, Jenny's story moves it close to the heart of what the NHS has always been about: a large-scale mechanism for generating social solidarity. Linking transparency to the natural desire to share one's stories with others gives us a system that can transmute private distress into public goods, at scale. Many more people can get involved, many more staff engaged, many more services improved.

29

Temptations of cheap data

Valerie Iles

Over the last 15 years, the capacity for data-holding and data-processing has increased hugely, and become very cheaply available. So, the ability to collect and compare data has become greater and more tempting.

One consequence of this is a 'culture of audit' (Strathern, 2000). It has had many beneficial outcomes, for example, focusing on healthcare based on evidence, highlighting inequalities in the take-up of healthcare across populations and identifying variations in performance between individuals, teams and organisations. Or, rather, audits and data comparisons identify variation in *aspects* of performance. This is an important distinction. Once upon a time – 20 years ago – those of us involved in the Resource Management Initiative were careful to point out that the purpose of information was not to provide answers (and certainly not judgements about performance), but to form the basis of a conversation, in the course of which – if well-managed and rigorously pursued – meaningful answers and sound judgements might emerge.

Since then, our ability to collect and compare data has fuelled our wish to reduce to code everything we possibly can, even where the code can reflect only part of a process we are interested in. For example, we collect data on what healthcare professionals do during a consultation with a patient, the decisions they reach and some of the factors they have considered, but very little about the ways in which they reached those decisions. This is understandable since decisions are often reached through an intuitive process involving tacit as well as explicit knowledge, not amenable to this kind of reduction to data. Unfortunately, our inability to do justice to complex situations through the data we collect has not been matched by a circumspection that would protect us from inappropriate uses of data.

Also fuelled by changes in information technology, our media have pandered to and promoted our desire to tell simple tales of fault and blame. They have reduced complex situations with many variables that interact in rich, unpredictable ways, in which some unhappy outcomes are inevitable. Resulting cries for accountability and transparency have found a receptive home in a style of management that likes to achieve results by 'holding people's feet to the fire', rather than purposeful, ongoing, direct conversations in which individuals are both supported and judiciously challenged in ways that meet their growing abilities as well as the situations they currently face.

Politicians have been affected by and have encouraged the demand for individual choice, failing to perceive – or choosing to ignore – that this comes at the expense of community value. They have introduced quasi-markets, choice and competition, backed up by a regulatory framework that can only access evidence on second-order processes rather than the care processes themselves.

All of this has increased hugely the amount of data that 'needs' to move around the system: so that performance can conform to specifications, so that audit trails can protect those offering and managing care, and so that consumers can make 'informed choices' between care providers. These massive amounts of data are also valuable to those wishing to go to litigation or encourage litigation, and the resulting increase in litigation costs prompts healthcare organisations to adopt lowest-risk options, even where there are good reasons for choosing paths with higher risks.

The care we so often want to give and receive has other aspects that look more like a relationship – a covenant – between care-giver and care receiver. We might conclude that it is the fault of policymakers and managers that data is being used to reduce our concept of healthcare to a set of auditable transactions in a marketplace. Contrasts between 'covenantal' and 'transactional' care are listed in the table at the end.

But we should also examine how we ourselves contribute to audit culture. If we wish to see the care offered in the NHS including good care transactions and also, when the occasion demands it, a covenant of care, we must examine some of our own behaviours and underlying assumptions. For example, when we hear of an unfortunate outcome, we might refrain from immediately demanding to know who is at fault. We might choose instead to acknowledge multiple factors at play, and design sensitive interventions that recognise the complexity. We might stop demanding accountability for delivering major changes in complex systems involving hundreds or thousands of people (like the 18-week target in hospitals) from individuals who cannot possibly influence all the relevant people and factors, and can only achieve it in ways that reduce the humanity, capability and resilience of the system.

We might recognise that when we audit anything, we are never merely observing what is happening. In the process of auditing, we are changing what happens. Sometimes this will have benefits that are worthwhile. Sometimes it will change behaviours in ways we would not want, for example, reducing creativity and increasing our aversion to risk. We might decide that there are other ways of finding out what it is we are interested in. Audit culture is only sometimes valuable.

We might stop taking an interest in simplistic league tables, and find other ways of accounting to the public for what we are doing with their healthcare money: giving sufficient weight to what matters to people, and not simply resorting to data that are readily collectible or can be mined from what is already held. We need ways of understanding what is happening that are as rich and complex as the situations they represent, and which require nuanced, thoughtful, judicious reflections rather than instant, computable 'answers'.

Just because we can place data alongside other data and come up with comparisons, which we may regard as answers or judgements, does not mean we should.

Covenantal and transactional care compared

Covenantal care	Transactional care
Healthcare with elements of the gift economy. Care that results from a relationship, a covenant, between care-giver and receiver.	Healthcare in the market economy. Patient as consumer, professional as provider.
Patient is cared about as well as for.	Patient is cared for.
Professionals recognise that in their encounters with patients, they give *and* receive.	Professionals are seen as givers (suppliers) of services.
Focus on thoughtful, purposeful judgement. This is necessarily subjective ('A view from somewhere'). It embraces objective measures and evidence.	Focus on calculation and counting. This can be seen as objective ('A view from nowhere').
Has emergent creativity, which can include the use of protocols.	Has predetermined protocols.
Wisdom and silence in addition to discourse and action.	Discourse and hyperactivity.
Tacit as well as explicit knowledge.	Explicit, formally codified knowledge.
Reflection on feelings and ethics as well as facts and figures.	Reflection on facts and figures.
Focus on the quality of the moment as well as efficiency and effectiveness.	Focus on efficiency and effectiveness.
Keeping in mind the meaning of the encounter for both parties while addressing the presenting problem.	Dealing with the presenting problem.
The humanity of the professional is also called upon, as well as competence.	Competence is what is called for on the part of the professional.
Individuals have a relationship with the community and with wider society.	Individuals have a relationship with the state and with the market.
Policy ideas can stay rich and be added to creatively, so that solutions are responsive, humane, practical, flexible, and adaptable. The focus is on solving problems.	Good policy ideas degenerate as they are translated at every level of the system into a series of measurable, performance manageable actions and objectives. The focus is on being able to demonstrate that policy has been implemented.

30

Overview: Innovation in cultures, feelings and roles

Mike Hales

This chapter looks at the challenges, and pressures and opportunities for innovation, that arise for professional and organisational cultures in healthcare via the constantly evolving potentials of information and communications technologies (ICTs). In reviewing the preceding seven contributions, it highlights six issues:

- Digital patient records can serve the well-being of self-caring service users in numerous ways. Different people tend to recognise different contributions to well-being.
- 'Cheap voice' arising from digital publication of users' comments is implicated in more than one kind of economics. Innovators have choices.
- Achieving engagement across 'colliding worlds' proves to be an internal issue as well as an external patient and public involvement (PPI) issue.
- Healthcare culture is challenged by the facilitation of dialogue.
- Healthcare culture is challenged by emerging ways of using and accessing data and documents.
- Cheap ICT solutions highlight a cultural conundrum: how much protocol is enough?

Finally, it offers some comments on how we might view innovation in this light: something that brings outcomes in 'technology'? Something that brings outcomes in culture, in feelings and in roles?

Digital patient records serve the well-being of self-caring service users in numerous ways

All three contributors concerned with personal information (Bennett, Fisher, Goldberg) are oriented to self-care – 'the fully engaged service user' and their well-being – but in different ways. As a service user, Yvonne Bennett highlights the possibility that some aspects of well-being may arise not from medical intervention using the data in the medical record, but from the records themselves, as resources that may help a person *tell a story*: making sense of their own life ('How I got my flat spine') and feeding into their concern with the lives of others they care about ('What my children need to look out for, in my grandchildren's health'). In contrast, as a GP, Brian Fisher is concerned with ways in which the medical record – as a rich, integrated, co-produced collation of personalised *data* – can facilitate engagement and dialogue between patients and medical practitioners as co-producers of care, 'live' in the consulting room. At the same time, he is aware that, as a publishing mechanism, the electronic patient record can also take the service into the patient's home, through novel extensions that provide links to documentary resources that a fully engaged service user may exploit in managing their own well-being outside the surgery.

Like Fisher, Lawrence Goldberg, as a hospital clinician, is oriented to data rather than stories. He brings a focus on engaging with individual patients to deliver care 'one patient at a time', not only through integrated personal data that is uniformly available in all healthcare settings (bridging the clinical silos of individual specialties), but also through facilities for analysing patterns in data in the consulting room. This can enable proactive responses that may make the difference, for example, between a patient with a long-term illness being able to stay at home and at work, managing their own health day to day in familiar settings, or having to go into hospital for urgent care.

Thus, numerous kinds of contributions to the well-being of the self-caring service user arise: resources for their story about themselves and their lives, for dialogues between healthcare professionals and service users, for self-care outside the consulting room and for 'joined-up' resources for service providers, accessible across medical silos and geographical distances. It is a simple point, but worth noting, that these different benefits tend to be 'naturally' recognisable for participants who are differently located in the process of healthcare (patients, GPs, hospital consultants, etc). This implies that to recognise and realise all benefits in innovative applications of ICTs, dialogues across these communities of practice are needed. Another point, easy to neglect, is that each of these insights into benefits, concerned in their own way with well-being and self-care, has its own quality of feeling (a mother for her family, a consultant with pride in his skilled team and their capacity for 'proactive' care, etc). As Ray Flux suggested in the closing paragraphs of his overview of Section 1, motivations to innovate arise from feelings, and go off in a particular direction because of this. Also, facilitation of dialogue involves working sensitively and skilfully with feelings – something touched on by Sims and Reed in Section 5.

Cheap voice, but more than one kind of economics

Rather than the live co-production of care, the contributors concerned with public information as user feedback (Taylor, Bacon, Hodgkin) address the offline context of service improvement, and are concerned with components of well-being that arise from choices that service users make outside the consulting room or hospital. It is something of a hygiene factor: when we are feeling bad, if we do not know where to turn for high-quality medical attention, we feel even worse. All three contributors address the potential of an economics of *cheap voice*, which is associated with the increasing ease of publishing documents (commentaries, ratings, etc) globally via online digital media.

Both Tris Taylor and Neil Bacon assert a service-consumer's perspective. Rather than the self-managing, fully engaged patient, in live dialogue with providers of care services (the focus for Bennett, Fisher and Goldberg), Taylor and Bacon show us the fully alert and assertive *consumer*, gathering market intelligence by cheaply mining cheaply published (though generally not quality-controlled) digital sources. In this context, individuals' experiences get codified (as digital story-texts, reviews, tags, star-ratings, etc) and shared through a process of digital goods being broadcast universally and consumed individually by other consumers. There is often no ongoing partnership or direct communication or interaction; it is a virtual marketplace. Bacon calls it 'enlightening the next user' and this function contributes to self-care in the classic, *caveat emptor* mode of market liberalism. This is probably close to what UK governments mean when they speak of choice in healthcare.

In this market/consumerist mode, service improvement is an optional extra; service providers may also, at their discretion, choose to exploit the broadcast, public postings as market intelligence. Taylor implies that individual medical professionals will be uncomfortable if they do not. Bacon draws the analogy between iWantGreatCare (iWantGreatCare, 2011) and TripAdvisor, a widely used ratings website in the hotel and travel services sector.

Paul Hodgkin, however, goes further. He points out that *mutuality* can be built on the same base of cheap public voice – still without direct communication between user and provider – via stories anonymously published at the service users' discretion, free of charge; but with an added (and added-cost) capacity for narrowcasting as distinct from indiscriminate broadcasting. Funded as a subscription service to healthcare providers, Patient Opinion establishes a population of service users (hospitals) committed to using the information feed in service improvement. The service facilitates this with back-office actions that selectively channel the feedback and tag it ('what is good', 'what could be improved', etc). Thus, in this service setting, we have not one, but two kinds of users – service users and NHS staff – mutually engaged with a collection of publicly published digital documents, and with a mutual expectation that stories may be acted on. Each day, the Patient Opinion home page (Patient Opinion, 2011) highlights this relationship; for example, on 14 February 2012: 'Who's listening to your stories? 36,165 stories told; 1,583 staff listening; 233 stories have led to changes.'

ICT-based service innovators exploiting cheap voice and user feedback have cultural-economic choices they can make. They can fall by default into the dominant consumerist, transactional frame, or they can articulate some other, innovative (mutualist) logic.

Achieving engagement across 'colliding worlds'

Lawrence Goldberg developed his chapter from the transcript of an interview. I started the interview expecting a significant case of user-led ICT system development – and, indeed, it is. But part-way through I began to understand that he and I were oriented to different communities of users. My mind was in 'PPI space', thinking of the NHS patient and public involvement agenda, and therefore I was listening for tales of patients' participation, and stories of how presentations of the life-stories of people with chronic kidney disease had been pivotal in system design. These challenges do indeed figure in Goldberg's account, but mainly as arenas for future work rather than as achieved outcomes and relationships at the present stage. My expectation that I would hear stories about patients' stories – like those told by Hodgkin, Taylor or Bacon in the patient feedback and service improvement context – was mistaken.

Celia Davies (Section 3) uses the notion of 'colliding worlds' to explore challenges that arise in different forms of involvement and engagement for service users and their advocates and helpers. I am using the term here to highlight a different but parallel reality. The 'user-led' success story in Goldberg's article turns out to be mainly one of developing cross-community and cross-location dialogues *within the professional landscape of the NHS* in order to enable medical personnel to deliver a joined-up service that parallels a patient's journey through the silos and sites of NHS departments and establishments. The numerous cultural worlds in these domains of practice – ward nurses, technicians, auxiliaries, hospital consultants, general practitioners, practice nurses, practice managers, line managers, accountants and others within the complex hierarchies of the medical world – are no less in collision than the worlds of NHS outsiders and insiders. It is not easy to develop and sustain an innovative focus on the diverse needs of these multiple communities of practice that need to be served by the system in order that the system's (insider) users can serve patients and their well-being.

With regard to innovation in patient-centred ICT tools and resources, Goldberg's case study demonstrates that the work of facilitating engagement – specifically, dialogue – across colliding cultural and professional worlds within the NHS is as central as the work of securing engagement, PPI-style, across the NHS–patient boundary.

Healthcare culture is challenged by the facilitation of dialogue

The challenges of developing and supporting the necessary dialogues are hard to meet. Goldberg suggests that the significant skills and insights needed to achieve this (Jane Keep addresses some of these in Section 3) may to some extent be counter-cultural. They are, at least, somewhat rare:

> We now understand that facilitation of dialogue or the design and execution of group processes are in themselves skills outside of the

usual clinical professional field, lying beyond the kinds of professional competencies typically found in the NHS.... Many clinicians and managers still find this foreign and 'soft'. (Goldberg, this section)

Innovating ICT systems and their usage involves a prolonged and complex process. Achieving a dialogue across silos and geographical locations, and sustaining the collective perspective through the process, is a challenge that demands skills more often associated with community development than healthcare. They cannot be taken for granted. Goldberg notes:

> The willingness to trust and engage in processes of learning and exploration across usual boundaries, which may be quite well known in 'the outside world' (like action learning), is not yet deeply embedded in our own culture. In furthering our project's aims for quality and integration, and the dialogues they depend on, I am not sure that we yet know where to look for these essential skills.

We might add that NHS managers and clinicians also find it hard to justify the spending that needs to be committed if full engagement (across boundaries either inside or outside the organisation) is to be supported by 'soft-skilled' professional facilitation, of the kind that Goldberg and his colleagues learned to value. This is significant work. Engagement does not just happen, and it is reasonable to expect that good-quality 'dialoguing' work will need to be paid for.

Healthcare culture is challenged by emerging ways of using and accessing data and documents

ICTs continually evolve under powerful market and cultural pressures. Attitudes and skills constantly emerge among communities of ICT use inside and outside the healthcare sector: users of mobile phones, personal computers, the internet, online purchasing, email and so on. Bacon and Taylor (regarding public information) and Fisher (regarding personal records) are in no doubt that because of developments in these areas, individual medical professionals will find themselves up against real challenges in their personal practice, and may find this medicine hard to take. (Celia Davies explores related aspects of what she calls *classic professional identity* in Section 5.) Bacon argues that: 'Perhaps in this case, rather than the doctor, it is the patient who knows best'. Taylor issues a direct challenge to medical professionals on behalf of patients: 'If you try to avoid making information available, I will find that suspicious'. And while Fisher is supportive and encouraging, he also notes that: 'This is a real information revolution, and a challenge for clinicians', which may lead them to feel that 'this is such a profound shift in the balance of forces that we should proceed, if at all, with great caution. Who knows what might happen if we [GPs] forgo our privileged access to this personal information [in the patient record]?'

At another level, with regard to *institutional forms and management cultures*, Hodgkin notes that cheap voice, cheap collaboration and the cost-free transport of digital commodities undermine the conventional economics of engagement and collaboration, creating an environment that the traditional culture of the NHS finds odd and hard to invest in. Hodgkin writes of a 'gift economy' and suggests that in the transactional world of NHS management and administration (a cultural reality that Valerie Iles is concerned with too; see later), gift-giving tends to be counter-cultural.

How much protocol is enough? And how are ICTs implicated?

Taylor and Bacon take for granted consumers' exploitation of ubiquitous cheap devices (phones and computers) and masses of cheap data in cyberspace. Hodgkin engages more critically with these facts of digital life and acknowledges that, for mutuality, additional back-office costs are involved if the value of narrowcasting rather than indiscriminate broadcasting is to be achieved by an ICT-based publishing service. Valerie Iles is more deeply critical of the culture that has arisen on the base of cheap data about the financial and medical performance of healthcare organisations and individuals. Alongside the apparent cheapness of ubiquitous data, and of performance metrics cheaply derived from these in real time and cheaply published, she is concerned that these resources are mundanely used in ways that are cheap in another sense. It is not just cost reduction, but also the devaluation of creativity and mature responsibility. While cost reduction is a core focus within NHS 'audit culture', it may be more accurate to say that management in the NHS has a deep (and understandable) orientation to *risk reduction*; and that a lot of money and emotional capital has been invested in an expectation that risk management might be made foolproof through a formidable array of auditable protocols combined with a massive evidence base.

Iles argues that around such an infrastructure of routinised protocol and cheap data and communication, there is a fundamental need for a highly developed ethos of responsible action and self-reflection among decision-makers of all kinds, grounded in a sense of mutual and empathetic rather than transactional relationships. She invites us to see that it is not just down to 'them' (Accountants? Managers?): we all are culpable for our willingness to do things the cheap and easy way, to tick audited boxes, and to fall back on (data) resources and standardised protocols just because they happen to be there in massive quantities.

Through this very human process, an audit culture has an innate tendency to degenerate into a 'jobsworth' regime in which the rock-bottom concern is to be able to demonstrate – through the audit trail – that what was done was what was contracted, specified or mandated by policy and protocol; and thus, to park elsewhere the blame for any harm (Iles, 2011). Rick Stern (Section 2) looked at this kind of behaviour in his discussion of senior managers' failures to take adequate responsibility on safety. He also outlined an experiment in which ICTs

– confidential digital publishing – are used to encourage and support reflective practice.

Iles' critique has some purchase not only on Taylor and Bacon's transactional perspective, but also on Fisher's argument for background information being automatically published via links to the patient record: standard documents, shipped according to standard protocols. Fisher notes how:

> messages about stopping smoking will be seen only by smokers – automated social marketing. Third parties will be able to create gadgets that automatically and securely use key data from the record to help you look after yourself better in a personalised and effective manner. (Fisher, this section)

It is hard to determine a point at which automated guidance might morph into Big Brother. It is not that an advocate of the automated, targeted, narrowcast publishing of documentary guidance – or even an advocate of helpful gadgets – is a Bad Person (manifestly untrue). Rather, it is that our tendency as both service providers and self-caring citizens to let protocols take over the work can be a primrose path to a lowered quality of relationships, attenuated empathy, a lessened sense of mutuality and responsibility – and, thus, to a lessened sense of well-being and selfhood. It is complicated. How much protocol is enough?

Innovation in technology? Innovation in cultures, feelings, roles

In this overview, I have chosen to look for challenges that arise for professional and organisational cultures in healthcare via the constantly evolving potentials of ICTs. It is through these cultures, and the visions and the gut feelings that they nurture and generate, that the potentials of data and digital media are exploited in actual innovations and made solid, not only through financial investment, but also through the emotional investments of users and managers. Innovators – in technology, in medical practice, in service management, in financial practice, in commissioning, in leadership, in engagement – have choices that they can make in which of their own feelings they work from, and which they facilitate through their work.

They may further enshrine individualism and transactional logic; they might evolve mutualism, a communitarian ethos and alliances in mutual welfare across communities of practice. They might feed a protocol-limited, jobsworth regime with more and more auditable, data-massive records systems; they might facilitate mature, negotiated, responsible, dialogue-based care-giving and risk-taking (by service providers and service users both) alongside skilled and informed use of the digital documents that make up the evidence base and the evolving patient records infrastructure.

In the current climate of suspicion over entrepreneurial GPs in the context of GP commissioning (*clinical commissioning*, as currently reframed), it is worth noting that an innovative and motivated (and appropriately trained) GP can also design a business model and marketing rationale for a service, free at the point of use, that promotes mutuality. Patient Opinion happened in this way (North West SHA, 2007; Social Innovation eXchange, 2008; Patient Opinion, 2011).

Leaders in healthcare need to offer leadership here. In large, hierarchical, multi-department, multi-site enterprises in the hospital sector, with layers of formal management, it may be conventionally obvious who those leaders should be. In the small-enterprise, general practice sector, it is harder to identify the locus of leadership (although the evolution of GP roles in commissioning frameworks looks interesting). And in the future, as public health (embedded in local government and the not-for-profit sector as well as the NHS) becomes relatively more important for the economy and for well-being, it gets really interesting – innovations in leadership just *have* to happen!

I am with Bob Sang in believing that, as a value, self-management applies not only to self-care by service users, but also *within* work communities in the NHS. However, self-management and creative, discretionary, responsible action are in tension with the heavily protocol-based and hierarchical modes of managerial accountability that over recent decades have assumed dominance within the NHS. Imagine a generation of managers, leading for self-management, mutualism and sustained engagement across colliding worlds inside and outside the NHS? Now *that* would be an innovation!

SECTION 5

What kind of learning, what kind of leadership?

Introduction

'Leadership' is cited as the magic ingredient when service improvement is under the microscope, and there are some pretty well worked models of how to develop leadership within organisations – and sometimes even across organisational boundaries. However, the literature has barely begun to get to grips with what it means to lead a health system predicated on placing people who use services at the centre. In discussing the rise of the patient leader, David Gilbert asked this question: '[W]here is the learning and support for such a blossoming of talent? Professional development is a well-recognised term after decades of investment in staff training. Learning and support for patient leaders is almost non-existent' (Gilbert, 2012b, p 1).

This section begins to scratch the surface of the question: what kind of leadership, if we are to achieve services shaped around co-creation and co-production? It opens with two context-setting chapters. Both wrestle with questions of continuity and change. **Alastair Mant** reminds us that the principles of good management are constant, even when contexts change dramatically. **Celia Davies** takes a retrospective look at the many-headed Hydra of the NHS, and the particular challenges of leading it in any form.

We then move to accounts of practice. A straightforward account by **Jon Willis**, a nurse, explains how listening to patients and relatives helped transform dementia care in his ward. **Kate Hall** writes of her own take on leadership as requiring the exercise of courage if patient and public interests are to remain at the forefront of organisational mindsets preoccupied with finance and regulation.

Moving back to the bigger picture, **Ed Nicol** and **Simon Eaton**, medical consultants working in the NHS, write about the rationale for and parameters of a co-productive health leadership model. **Simon Duffy**, one of the original architects of individual budgets, reflects on what we can learn from history in learning disability, a field that has been seeking to practice co-creation approaches for a quarter of a century. He points out that none of the major steps forward have come from the top; all have been pushed by people working and campaigning from outside the system – families, disabled people, academics and activists. **Malik Gul** then describes how people who are usually regarded as hard to reach by services can become a resource (and resourceful) rather than a challenge when formal services get out there and talk with them. The objective is to 'bend the mainstream' so that it can serve all in a respectful and effective way.

These overviews are followed by two contributions that explore specific applications in the context of development programmes. Sometimes a perspective from elsewhere can prompt reflection that frees up ideas for improvements: **Ian Cunningham** draws on experience in the education sector, supporting head teachers to develop person-centred approaches within their schools, through self-managed learning. He reiterates the importance of intangibles – values, vision and moral purpose – for credible and sustainable leadership. **Tim Sims** and **Fiona Reed** address two themes that are essentials in the leadership toolkit: appreciative enquiry (learning from what is right rather than what is wrong) and facilitation of dialogue. Finally, editor **Jan Walmsley** reflects on lessons from the section, and some gaps to fill, for those who seek to understand what leadership means in the world envisioned by the book's contributors.

31

Managers and leadership, now and then

Alastair Mant

The Griffiths Report into management of the NHS was published almost 30 years ago (Griffiths Report, 1983). At the time, many health professionals were sceptical about a supermarket boss having anything useful to say about the provision of professional services in a nationalised setting. Griffiths' big idea was that nobody was really in charge of anything in the 'consensus' or 'matrix' organisation of the health service. Following Griffiths, managers were introduced to (or imposed upon) the service.

Management then

The Prime Minister of the day, it is worth remembering, believed that big business held all the answers and that public services were irredeemably old-fashioned and inefficient. In no time at all, the new managers were installed as the villains of the piece in the minds of many health service workers – and especially in the minds of the doctors. I remember saying to Sir Len Peach, seconded from IBM as personnel head and then chief executive, "If the managers really have to have cars in their incentive package, make a rule that nobody gets a BMW!" I was too late, even if I was taken seriously.

What did we mean by management back in 1983 and what do we think it is today? Has the managerial job changed as a result of new technologies for example? Griffiths wrote his report just at the moment when 'management' began to be supplanted by 'leadership' in the discourse of organisational life. It seemed that managers, Peter Drucker's heroes of the hour, were not good enough any more – we needed something more admirable: leaders.

Management now

Scroll forward to 2011 in order to examine what has happened to the actual practice of management in this brave new world. Choose a successful organisation that did not exist when Griffiths was published in 1983 – and which could not have been imagined then. Let's say, Google – founded in 1998 and currently market capitalised at US$171bn. Obviously, Google is a new kind of company, operating in a new kind of market inconceivable 27 years ago. Obviously, Google must be practising management in an entirely new kind of way. Or is it?

Helpfully, Google have done the research for us and very thoroughly indeed, as you might expect of the world's best data-miners. And they have kindly published the results under the rubric of Project Oxygen. They laboriously analysed thousands of performance reviews, feedback surveys, top-manager awards and exit interviews – any data they could get their hands on – and submitted the results to a search-engine-style correlation of words and phrases. Google statisticians gathered more than 10,000 manager observations across 100 variables and then sat down to read everything and to discuss, argue and make judgements about what their employees were telling them.

The outcome? A list of eight qualities that Google employees wished more of their bosses possessed, and the last of these in importance was technical capability. It turned out that everybody values bosses who are 'even-keeled', who make time for one-on-one meetings, who help subordinates to puzzle through problems by asking smart questions, and who take a serious interest in employees' lives and careers. They summarised findings under three heads:

- Have a clear vision and strategy for the team's work (*My boss is smart*).
- Help your employees with career development (*My boss cares*).
- Do not be a sissy; be productive and results-oriented (*My boss is decisive*).

Above all, it seems that the good boss always keeps the value-added outcomes of the service in the forefront, not just the outputs or, in the modern world, the 'targets' imposed from above.

Homer Simpson might observe: 'D'oh!' And had Homer existed in 1983, it would have been just the same: 'D'oh!' Some things do not change. It seems that the good boss still thinks straight, relates well and acts powerfully.

32

Harnessing a Hydra – managing to change the NHS

Celia Davies

Today's quest for more leadership in the NHS makes me uneasy. I am less uneasy now that we are not hailing the heroes of the battlefield but focusing instead on distributed leadership, servant leadership and related concepts. But I am still concerned. A career in social research has left me with a strong conviction that the concepts we use matter. I am often reminded of the old adage about the drunk and the lamp post. We use concepts for support rather than illumination. Much talk of leadership, I believe, exhorts more than it illuminates. It directs attention away from some fundamentals.

To manage the NHS in a locality is to face three directions at once. There is *managing upwards* – having an eye to changing policy and regulatory demands, interpreting the opportunities as well as the constraints. There is *managing outwards* – much has been said in Sections Two and Three of this book about involving multiple stakeholders from the community in service design and evaluation. And there is *managing inwards* – a large part of which, but by no means all, involves relating to the work of the professions of medicine and nursing. In periods of observing the NHS intermittently over a career of 40 years and more as a social researcher, I have kept coming back to the social relations between the doctor, the nurse and the manager.

A hesitant start

I published my first academic paper in 1972 on professionals in organisations. A fresh-faced young sociologist, I had assimilated Max Weber on the positives of bureaucratic organisation compared with charismatic or autocratic rule – the reliability of rule-following, the progressive accommodation of a bigger picture level by level and the political direction at the top. I had read about bureaucracies in practice, however, and had devoured Robert Merton's classic concept of 'trained incapacity', the notion that the capacity of the bureaucrat – vital in some circumstances – was dysfunctional in others. I had also studied professions – individual accountability and the need for autonomy in the practice of expertise were at the heart of this concept. Professionalism seemed the very antithesis of bureaucratic rule-following, and conflict between professionals and bureaucrats seemed the inevitable consequence.

A glimpse of what this might mean on the ground came from a first foray into fieldwork in a small London hospital. Sitting in the office of the then hospital secretary, circulars from the Ministry covering the desk, he explained that the door would regularly burst open and demands from the senior medical staff would follow. "Sometimes when I go home," he mused, "I wonder whether I should consult with the worms before I cut the grass." Peace-making and troubleshooting were a large part of his activity. Years later, when one study was to dub managers as 'diplomats' (Harrison and Lim, 2003), the concept had immediate resonance with me. Later still, the concept of a bureau-professional regime underpinning the creation of the welfare state emerged (Clarke and Newman, 1997). Faith in the professions ran high – the role of the state was providing the conditions where new medical interventions could be deployed as widely as possible for the population.

Later came the chance to spend time observing doctors in their daily work with patients, in their deeply hierarchical relations with juniors and also in the hospital's medical committees. The agenda for one meeting included an item on priorities for development. Speeches were made. "Gentlemen," said the Chair, "we must not be parochial." These doctors were deeply individualistic and non-corporate. They had daily encounters with grateful patients; their strong sense of personal confidence and responsibility ('I carry the can') frequently spilled over into arrogance. Years later, reading the minutes of some British Medical Association (BMA) meetings, I again detected the challenge of generating commitment to collective positions. Later still, I read of a doctor who had contacted a registrant to say he disagreed with the General Medical Council (GMC) panel decision of which he had been part. I was to make more of this lack of corporate loyalty much later.

Nursing didn't fit!

What of nurses? The sociology of the 1970s offered me the concept of a semi-profession – aspiring to full professional status but not there yet. But there was more. Nurses were railing against the role of handmaid to the doctor and struggling to produce what today is called patient-centred care. Their expertise was contested and difficult to demonstrate with a labour force in hospitals comprised of trainees, transient bank nurses and those in assistant grades. Like a would-be full profession, they aspired to stronger educational criteria for entry, but the job of the qualified nurse was largely not to nurse herself but to supervise others. It also fell to nurses to coordinate care. As late as the mid-1990s, a colleague fresh from observation on a hospital ward came back to report that the nurses had a string of yellow sticky post-its on their arms, reminding them to find missing notes, locate a junior doctor, chase a test and so on. I wrote at one point about 'coping management' as widespread.

It took me many years – and the arrival of feminist theory – before I was to make the suggestion that nursing was not so much a 'semi-profession' as an adjunct to a profession. Ensuring the right people and the right information were in place at the right time, and mopping up tears and fears, enabled doctors to appear and depart, to utilise their expertise in a 'fleeting encounter'. There was an uncomfortable contradiction for nursing in trying to create a profession out of an adjunct to a profession (Davies, 1995). At the time, I stressed the hidden work of caring more than what was also represented by those yellow stickies – the hidden work of management.

Classic professional identity and two sequelae

Two points arise from this. One has to do with the preservation of what I came to call classic professional identity (CPI; see following box). Like the bureaucratic personality, it is not meant to characterise each and every individual, but rather to accentuate tendencies. Like the bureaucratic personality too, it has a downside. Most obviously, it can create arrogance and failure to acknowledge the work of others. Less obviously, it raises expectations and makes unrealistic demands for a cure, as doctors themselves sometimes acknowledge (West, 2004). It also, however, creates blind spots about the value of being managed in a supportive way and about the knock-on effects and costs of actions taken solely with the individual patient in view. Attention to the most obvious of these features brought me a bad press with some in the profession and an accusation that I was living in the days of the 'Carry On' film character Sir Lancelot Spratt.

Classic professional identity (CPI)

•	A strongly bounded individual	*A sense of self apart from others*
•	Mastery of knowledge	*Expertise as a hard-won personal acquisition*
•	Detachment	*Emotionally controlled and self-referential*
•	Autonomous practice	*A unilateral, personally accountable decision-maker*
•	Interchangeability	*A 'company of equals' with presumed equal competence*
•	A singular identity	*Professional identity outweighs/transcends other identities*

Source: Davies (2003)

There is a further point. Immense commitment frequently accompanies both CPI and adjunct professionalism. Doctors return in off-duty time, nurses stay at the end of the shift, managers take work home, clinics and surgeries overrun. The work is still managed in large measure around the patient's encounter with the doctor. And it is accomplished through coping more than active management – sometimes despite systems (which can be multiple, contradictory and overlapping) rather than because of them.

Towards today

For those inclined to dismiss all this as extreme or out of date, consider this. A series of improvement projects was carried out in one of the highest-status NHS Foundation Trusts in London in 2010/11. What to an outsider surely looks extraordinary is how seemingly 'unmanaged' the different service areas were. Referrals were duplicated, patients were booked into the wrong clinics, bottlenecks and long clinic waits were common, theatre use was low with frequent list order changes and late starts, records were made in multiple forms and were often lost, equipment was missing, and so on. (A related phenomenon is hinted at too in Goldberg's discussion of fragmentation to be overcome with patient records, see Section 4.) One of the service managers tells an inspiring story of hurdles overcome and changes made (Nyadzayoo, 2011). Similarly inspiring but again basic improvement work is documented in the work of the NHS Institute for Innovation and Improvement (www.institute.nhs.uk). There may be more computers these days but the yellow-sticky world is still alive.

Things have changed. A fuller story would need to cover the changing composition of the health professions, the emergence of organised patient groups and the breakdown of relations of deference that underpinned the social organisation of healthcare described here. With props to the old regime crumbling, it would need to explore why – more than a decade after an acknowledgement that the NHS needed to modernise and the unprecedented increases in investment, when austerity started to bite – patients were still experiencing delays and staff were still running fast to stay in the same place.

Importantly, the NHS is awash with transformation leads and service improvement projects. These are demonstrating just what can be achieved when people pause and come together to analyse how they have been working, what it means for patients and where the costs fall. Projects, however, are immensely fragile. There has to be the clout to assemble the group and the facilitated time to bond and work together. Skills to track and represent outcomes in ways that will ensure sustainability locally are vital. Unintended consequences abound – new targets and tariffs from on high, for example, can push service improvements off course. Interestingly, the King's Fund brought management into the title of its recent leadership commission and emphasised its importance throughout (King's Fund, 2011).

To lead change in healthcare is to struggle with the many-headed Hydra that is the NHS. It is to engage with the committed and the clever, whose focus, understandably, is more often on healthcare interventions than on the organisation of those interventions. But to return to the opening remarks, it also means more than looking inward. Change-makers at all levels have the task of interpreting the policy regime and delineating, and then monitoring, the space it allows for positive change. They need to be in dialogue with patients and the public – not just explaining change, but giving people the chance to participate in shaping that change. The question is: are our current concepts and understandings of leadership robust enough for the job?

33

"Ask the patient what they want"

Jon Willis

I met Bob Sang when I applied for a place on the Health Foundation Leadership scheme. I wasn't quite sure what to make of him at first. He looked a bit like a social worker or geography teacher but his ideas and thoughts challenged much of what I took for granted. Before being 'Bobbed', as a nurse, I used to do what I thought best for the patient. Now I ask them. Such a simple change has had a profound effect on the care we provide on the ward.

When I took over the running of a 28-bedded care of the elderly ward, it felt as though Bob was sitting on my shoulder whispering: "Ask the patient what they want." That is what I did, in a very unscientific way. I talked to patients, relatives, carers and went out into the community to a number of dementia cafes. These were chastening experiences. I was told in no uncertain terms where the Trust was going wrong.

I was embarrassed by what I heard. The ward routine was for the benefit of the staff not the patients. Patients were being woken at 5:30am to have observations done. Nutritional support was erratic, relatives were excluded except at visiting time and not included in care. There was nothing for the patients to do on the ward, they were bored.

Over the last two years, we have made great strides. Patients are no longer woken at the crack of dawn. Before the start of every shift, patients who need assistance with eating or drinking are identified at a safety briefing. They are provided with a red tray ensuring everybody is aware of their needs. Specialist crockery was purchased to help patients with dementia or reduced dexterity.

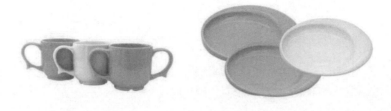

Relatives and carers are encouraged to come in to provide support or assistance at meal times and are welcome anytime. New signs with pictures have been put up.

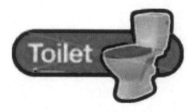

The Red Cross provide hand massages and 'the pat dog' is a weekly visitor. A local charity has funded live music on the ward. The effect on a number of patients has been remarkable. The musicians comment on the contented expressions on people's faces after they have played.

As a result of talking at the dementia cafes, we have developed a fantastic relationship with the Alzheimer's Society. They are funding £20,000 for an organiser to recruit and manage volunteers to help with patients on the ward. We have obtained funding for a flat-screen TV, computer, webcam and microphone. This will allow patients to communicate with relatives via Skype and will be used as a video box.

We are trying to find ways to get real uncensored and timely feedback. I am sure that having patients telling us what they really think will be a powerful tool that Bob Sang would approve of.

34

The heart and art of leadership

Kate Hall

I am known by those who work with me for saying what needs to be said, even when it is likely to be unpopular. I have no idea how I acquired this skill or how I developed it. I was once quite shy. What I do know is that I have a very strong inner sense of right and wrong, which means that I get my knickers in a twist if I see or sense injustice or unfairness and am then driven to do or say something. I used to try to conform to the masses – putting my head down for 'an easy life' – but I just couldn't do it. The number of times my inner voice used to say: "Don't say it, don't say it right now, it will go down really badly, just keep quiet and raise it later." But then I'd hear the words coming out of my mouth. After a while, I stopped even trying to keep quiet and decided that as I had this commitment to fighting injustice, I needed to use it.

Patients are people and should not be defined by their illness or diagnosis, but they often are. Patients are someone's mum, grandpa, dad, sister, daughter, son; they have needs, feelings, hopes and aspirations, as we all do, they just happen to be temporarily poorly, living with a long-term condition or reaching the end of their life.

I have felt for some time that those of us who have reached the dizzy heights (whatever they are) of NHS management do not always focus on patients in day-to-day work. Yes, of course policy is important and has its place, as does strategy and operational management, but policy, strategy and operational management are supposed to be for the good of the patient, not the convenience of people who work in the system.

I was challenged to refine my thinking on our duty as senior NHS professionals to put patients' interests first when I applied to become a Health Foundation Leadership Fellow in 2003. Bob Sang, whose work inspired this book, was a member of the team delivering the scheme. He always ensured that the patient was either physically or virtually in the room with us and at the centre of our discussions. He recruited Patient Quality Advisors, patients or relatives of patients, some of whom were living with long-term conditions, some of whom had been or continued to be users of the service. Their role was to bring 'the patient' into the room, to challenge our thinking face to face.

It took me quite a bit of time to get used to having patients involved; often, they were supportive of our efforts and ideas, but they also challenged hard; at times, they irritated us; at times, you could say that their comments were almost inappropriate; and, at times, they didn't understand what we were trying to achieve or why something was important – but what I didn't realise at the start, but came to appreciate through the process, was the significant difference they made.

Bob influenced me to always remember the patient, and that real patient involvement and working in co-production is crucial. We should not be irritated by patients or view them as a bit of a hindrance; but often people do, although they will never admit it. Patient involvement is not, and should not, simply be a 'tick-box' exercise or 'just enough'.

We all have a choice and my choice is to stand by my ideals no matter what, even though they might be unpopular. I generally speak out if I feel I need to, even when it is uncomfortable, which it often is, even when I might be the sole voice and even when it might make me unpopular and possibly labelled as 'trouble'. Having the ability to do it is one thing, it doesn't mean my skin is any thicker than anyone else's. Sometimes there are consequences and these can hurt, but when I get stuck over whether to say something or not, I find myself asking: "What is the right thing to do?". And then I get on and do it and worry about the consequences later. Right does not necessarily mean easy and right does not necessarily mean popular.

I continually remind myself and my colleagues that, as 'leaders', we must not lose focus on what or for who we are leading. I generally start presentations I give now with a slide saying 'Patients have a right to effective, safe care at all times'. I say it and then I wait. I then say that patients are our mother, brother, sister, grandpa, son, daughter or whoever, and that whenever we are talking about the health service, we should think about the standards that we would want for our families and friends. This seems to get people's attention (particularly when I am talking about something financial) and then, when I feel I've waited long enough, I get on with whatever I'm talking about and to whichever audience. Everyone needs reminding of this, no one is too senior.

My current role is less operational. I work alongside boards and focus on board development. I talk about quality daily and when presenting, I ask board members to consider three questions:

- How does the Board ensure that patient satisfaction and patient care are as important as financial and performance targets?
- What is the evidence that the Board gives the same attention to quality as that which is focused on finance?
- How does the Board ensure that patients and their experience are at the heart of the organisation's work?

I then ask them to add the word 'really' after 'does the Board'.

I'm sure there is more that I could do and writing this has refocused my mind. This is not about calling yourself a leader, having a swanky title, a good salary and 'power'. This is about holding on to personal values, passion, being able to deal with uncomfortable issues and courage. It is hard, but no one said leadership was easy.

35

Health leadership for the 21st century – a new, holistic, co-productive endeavour

Ed Nicol and Simon Eaton

Writing as NHS consultants, we put forward here a health leadership model recently published in the *Journal of the Royal Society of Medicine* (Nicol and Sang, 2010). It encompasses a clinical and a citizen/user perspective and is premised on the belief that if the NHS is to survive, health leadership must now be a co-productive endeavour between health workers, like ourselves, and patients, working within and beyond traditional NHS boundaries.

The article links the themes of sustainability – argued so convincingly in the Wanless report (Wanless, 2002); quality – the heart of Lord Darzi's report (Department of Health, 2008); and co-creative learning and development. It proposes a leadership model that offers an alternative to current public service models (Sang, 2009).

The authors believe that the NHS must always, as a minimum, provide safe maternity services; robust and timely emergency services; provide care to those with long-term conditions, looking to enable quality of life, not just quantity of life; and provide for a dignified end to life. However, it is clear that we cannot afford to provide for every possible eventuality and keep the NHS funded as it is. Patients and the wider public need to be engaged with clinicians in an open and frank debate about resource utilisation in a cash-limited NHS. Together, we must accept that tough and uncomfortable decisions are required and be willing to accept joint responsibility for these decisions, even when counter to potential vested interests. A wider view is required to ensure a broad continuous improvement in healthcare, based on reducing inequality and enabling a high-quality experience for all.

The greatest cost burden falls to supporting those with long-term conditions and it is here that we should focus our attention on changing the mindset and embracing a co-created system, with clinicians and patients working and learning together. 'Engagement', and its corollary 'empowerment', can no longer remain as easily misunderstood rhetoric, or marginalised as a patient and public involvement (PPI) function: they are core to leadership success throughout health and social care.

Providing safe, high-quality local services, including treatment for sickness and injury and effective, sympathetic social care, while also reducing inequalities and improving health and quality of life, is a hugely challenging and complex task. It requires health leaders, like ourselves, to meaningfully engage with all stakeholders throughout the whole cycle of commissioning and delivery.

The core relationship between clinicians and patients must evolve and take central place, not just at an individual consultation level, but on a wider, more strategic level. Together, they must both learn that effective healthcare is a joint endeavour: from diagnosis and clinical intervention, to supporting successful recovery and, most importantly, sustainable, independent living. The medical profession must desist from its all-too-familiar paternalism. Crucially, the NHS needs to move from simply collecting feedback to engaging patients and the public in prioritising, designing and delivering improved services.

Quality is a concept interpreted differently by users, clinicians and managers. A technically competent and evidence-based treatment pathway may provide clinical quality against recommended standards but does not necessarily define a quality experience for the user, and too often we, as providers, let ourselves down by allowing a lack of humanity and caring to persist in the system. Artificial boundaries between primary, secondary and social care, with conflicting incentives and separate budgets, often lead, at best, to an inefficient system and, at worst, to an ineffective and frustrating one, in which the user passes between agencies with little joined-up thinking or support. 'Quality' is an expression of public value that enriches people's lives and that, crucially, enhances where and how we live and work. It is the users of the service who should decide what quality is, and it is for this reason that including patient or service-user leadership is essential in a co-productive *health leadership* model.

The future sustainability of the NHS is dependent on wider public engagement and enhanced service productivity. The leadership required for active and successful engagement goes well beyond the traditional silos of clinical or managerial leadership and requires a holistic health leadership approach.

Patients are often better informed, less deferential and rightly more demanding than they once were, yet they still trust the medical profession (Bechel et al, 2000). The term 'patient' no longer feels appropriate to many with long-term conditions; paternalistic approaches are rejected by many. Clinicians too often fail to recognise the expertise of the individual and their families with regard to how the condition fits into their lives or their ideas about how to address it. Clinicians also need to remember and accept that there is robust evidence to show that improvements in satisfaction, safety, clinical outcomes and adherence to treatments often arise when patients take ownership of their own healthcare needs (Bechel et al, 2000; Garcia-Alamino et al, 2010; Brewis and Fitzgerald, 2011; Health Foundation, 2011).

Holistic, inclusive health leadership requires a different set of skills and attitudes than those required to lead a clinical team. As 'clinical leaders', we are increasingly entrusted with crossing professional boundaries and delivering cost-effective personalised healthcare. However, there are risks with advancing today's clinicians into different, more holistic future roles. Training programmes, particularly of doctors, have often focused on developing confidence and autonomy to make decisions in the face of uncertainty, often without recourse to others (see Davies on classic professional identity [CPI], this section). Our own learning about leadership indicates that clinicians must learn to develop a more collaborative and less directive approach to healthcare decisions, recognising the contributions of others, and understanding when our role should be facilitator, navigator or coach, rather than didactic expert.

Clinicians also need to embrace management involvement in the delivery of healthcare, rather than undermining it. Health managers must equally play their part. When management goals are expressed as improvement to clinical services (rather than in raw metrics), there is proven improvement in clinical outcomes and quality of services (Chief Medical Officer, 2009). Using plain English is vital to the successful engagement of clinicians, patients and carers, and should be a fundamental skill for any practising clinician or health manager. Multidisciplinary training and interaction between clinicians and managers should start early and continue throughout both career pathways, so that a mutual respect and trust can be built and the current misplaced apprehension and stereotyping challenged and overcome.

Wanless's 'fully engaged' scenario applies equally to clinicians as to wider society. Without an appreciation of the broadest definition of health, and the needs of the local healthcare economy, a clinician cannot be truly a healthcare leader.

Health delivery traditionally encompasses four domains: clinical, managerial, user and governmental (see following figure). Clinicians and patients are the recipients of a policy-driven agenda, with targets used to drive productivity and 'quality' while providing a basis for measuring outcomes – but not necessarily health improvement.

The domains of health leadership

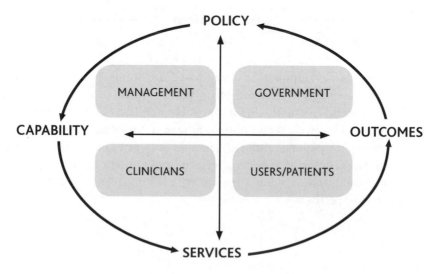

Source: Sang (2009).

Health improvement should be a matter of co-production and mutual learning (Cowper et al, 2004) – 'No decision about me, without me'. The co-productive health leadership model (see following figure) encompasses and supports this fully, and integrates a much higher involvement of users, building on projects such as the Expert Patients' Programme. This supports a more patient–led service with shared decision-making and accountability at all levels.

'The co-productive health leadership model'

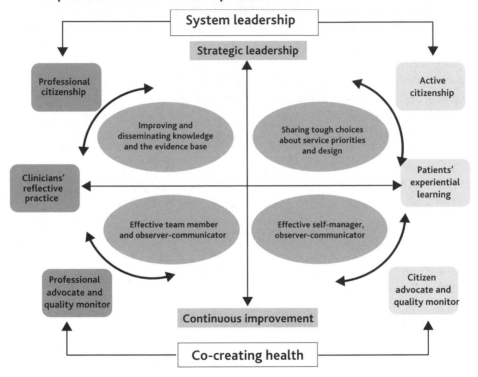

Conventional service development has been based on 'doing unto others', most recently by use of the integrated care pathway. This 'systematic and evidence-based design principle' should ensure the highest possible standard of clinical outcome for people with specific medical conditions. However, there is potential to limit personal ownership for patients, and the principle does not guarantee a 'quality' experience. Pathways describe the way a service or organisation aims to address a specific health issue or issues, but a person with a long-term condition does not live on a disease pathway.

Diabetes Year of Care

The Diabetes Year of Care programme has transformed people's experience of the consultation, putting them firmly in the driving seat of their care and supporting them to self-manage more effectively. Key products of the programme relating to personalised care planning included:

- a process by which people with diabetes attending for their annual review had their tests completed and results sent to them prior to their consultation;
- clinician training to support adopting a partnership approach, identifying an individual's goals and co-producing an action plan; and
- articulation of the 'whole system' infrastructure requirements to support this.

People with diabetes were central to all aspects of design and delivery of the programme, including formal and informal qualitative feedback as members of the local implementation teams, and in focus groups or other consultative events, to discuss specific issues or questions.

For more details, see: www.diabetes.nhs.uk/year_of_care

To take forward this agenda, health leaders, clinicians and citizens, commissioners and providers, all need to come together in flexible productive partnerships; sharing knowledge and experience, energy and enthusiasm, doubt and uncertainty. Our suggested *health leadership* framework aims to combine professional initiative and active citizenship. It incorporates clinicians' reflective practice but is equally informed by insights from patients' experiential learning. Used together, this would improve the clinician's insight into what is required to develop a 'quality' service from the user perspective, and the user would gain greater understanding of the challenges and limitations within the system. This approach requires clinicians and services not only to constantly seek out user feedback and ideas for improvement, but also to share responsibility for the prioritising, design and delivery of improvements with service users and the wider community (Boyle and Harris, 2011; Year of Care, 2011b).

Bengali cookery

Faced with the challenge of encouraging healthy eating among Bengali men with diabetes, Social Action for Health, a community development charity in Tower Hamlets, worked with local communities to set up a cookery club. Traditionally, Bengali men would not be involved in cooking and were not familiar with healthy eating messages. Using existing community leaders and networks, they recruited community workers, employed a local chef and used a kitchen in a community centre. By keeping it local and delivering the sessions from within the community, they have been able to engage this hard-to-reach group with healthy lifestyle messages.

See: 'Education sessions for people with diabetes'. Available at: www.towerhamlets.nhs.uk/news/diabetic-education-sessions

Patients and the wider public need to be engaged with clinicians in an open and frank debate about resource utilisation in a cash-limited NHS. Together, we must accept that tough and uncomfortable decisions are required, and be willing to accept joint responsibility for these decisions, even when they run counter to potential vested interests. A wider view is required to ensure a broad continuous improvement in healthcare, based on reducing inequality and enabling a high-quality experience for all. This model incorporates a grounded, iterative process of mutual engagement: both professional experts and experts by experience.

This approach to learning and development, if adopted, should support the NHS to become a system designed to promote health and well-being, and inform both commissioners and providers, who are open to being fully engaged with their users and wish to deliver a truly patient-informed healthcare system. Co-designed services facilitate individual care planning, still rightly informed by the traditional medical model, but accommodating individual needs, preferences and circumstances and enabling the NHS deliver a higher-quality service: personally, locally and systemically.

We must all embrace a wider health leadership responsibility. The central clinician–patient relationship must be retained at the core and clinicians must fight for patients' rights, not acquiesce and blame the system when it is too challenging. Clinicians must work collaboratively to develop a more co-productive, rewarding and cost-effective system. Dr Colin-Thomé recognised this requirement when reviewing the failings of Mid Staffordshire NHS Trust:

> Patient empowerment is a theme throughout my review, and I hope my recommendations in relation to patient empowerment are taken to heart by the NHS.... Patients must be involved in the design, delivery, and quality assurance of their services and ... clinicians must speak up for patients when they witness poor quality care. It is our overarching duty. (Colin-Thomé, 2009, p 7)

The sustainability of the NHS lies in changing the basis of the relationship between patients, clinicians and managers by adopting an adult–adult relationship based on equality, openness, informed dialogue and critical friendship. These are the key elements of co-productive 'health leadership' and these are the fundamental pillars that will determine the success of the NHS. As doctors, we look forward to playing our part.

36

Forty years of innovation in community responses to the needs of people with learning difficulties

Simon Duffy

Sometimes we imagine that we live in a rationally organised world where the best and the brightest are in power and that they will use their good will and intelligence to bring about beneficial social change. This powerful and dangerous illusion is called meritocracy.

The illusion of meritocracy is possible because we want to believe that the powerful know what they are doing and that they have our best interests at heart. Of course, this illusion also serves the powerful. This doesn't mean that the powerful are stupid or malicious. The reality is that our leaders are just as confused by the bewildering complexity of the modern world as the rest of us. But we pay them to behave as if they understand what is going on and are able to do something about it.

The meritocratic illusion often corrupts our understanding of history. Often, we uncritically accept that positive change is led by government. However, if we examine the detailed history of social change, we can see that government is not the leader, but the follower.

The end of the 20th century saw some progress for people with learning difficulties. They were able take some important steps to achieving active citizenship and overcoming prejudice and exclusion. One of the most important signs of progress was the closure of all long-stay hospitals or institutions. This process began in the 1970s when the institutions were at their peak size, and was finished in England in 2009 with closure of Orchard Hill Hospital in Surrey.

This process certainly involved government, but it was not begun by government. At least three things were needed in order to achieve this progress. First, progress demands some positive vision for an alternative reality and this largely came from the international movement called *normalisation*, inspired by independent thinkers like Wolf Wolfensberger. These thought leaders both provided a powerful critique of the failure of institutional models and offered a theory that seemed an attractive basis for developing a new way forward.

Second, this vision had to be brought to life with real and practical examples of positive change. In the UK, this movement took a particular form and books like *An ordinary life in practice* (Towell, 1988), with its description of models and good practice, helped to provide a different pattern. This phase was also marked by the increased cooperation and collaboration of thought leaders and practitioners as they tried to take people down this new path. Organisations like the Campaign for Mental Handicap grew up and provided a powerful voice for change.

Over time, the change process itself began to be normalised. Government was persuaded to develop the 'dowry system' – a way of moving funding out of NHS hospitals in to community services. This funding was combined with 'board and lodging funding', which lasted from 1980 to 1992 and subsidised the provision of residential care. Some NHS managers led the process of change, others resisted the change. Eventually, when most hospitals were already closed, it took a much more directive approach from government to complete the final closures.

The process of deinstitutionalisation did not just have to overcome the normal unwillingness to change that is found in every human being, it also had to overcome the power of vested interests and their ability to exercise political power in order to retain the status quo.

Innovations tend to follow a pattern, known as the diffusion of innovation curve. However, it is important to note that the shape of the innovation curve in public services is not identical to the normal curve that would be expected in commerce and industry. The following figure describes the diffusion of innovation in public services and the different patterns of resistance to innovation that are faced at each stage.

'The diffusion of innovation in public services'

© Simon Duffy

This curve varies from the normal curve because:

- Public services have little incentive to innovate and so innovations take much longer to be accepted.
- When government embraces an innovation, there is often a very quick take-up, although during this process, the innovation is often diluted in order to achieve the political goal.

- After formal political success has been achieved, government attention stops, this can then lead to a period of stagnation or delay.

In other words, public services tend to be immune to innovation and when innovations are backed by policymakers, this can often mask deeper problems of definition and implementation. The fact that the government has the power to declare something a success, despite the actuality, can sometimes lead to very shallow change.

We can see this pattern of resistance to innovation not just in the process of deinstitutionalisation, but also in the development of a more recent innovation: *personalisation*. Personalisation built upon social innovations like normalisation and independent living. For example, many people with learning difficulties who left hospital found that while they were living 'in the community', they still lacked all the normal levels of control and independence that make community living worthwhile. People found themselves with no control over who they lived with, who supported them or what they did each day. Instead, they discovered that institutionalisation could still survive within the confines of residential care homes, day centres and the underpinning systems of social work, funding and commissioning.

Today, it may seem obvious to most that in order to bring about positive change in people's lives, it would also be necessary to: (a) individualise funding; and (b) give people control over that funding. However, early innovators who advocated these ideas were largely ridiculed and excluded from policy discussions. Successful piloting of these ideas in Southwark in the early 1990s or in Glasgow in the late 1990s did not lead to any interest or discussion within policy circles.

The shift towards some kind of policy acceptance began in 2003 with the launch of the In Control pilot project in Wigan. This project was specifically designed to minimise some of the more predictable forms of resistance. In particular, the leaders of the project decided to:

- *Offer a positive vision for change* – The project combined a focus on new technologies (individual budgets, self-directed support and resource allocation systems) with attention to values, theory and the historical context of the changes.
- *Develop a strong and attractive brand* – Instead of treating the pilot as an academic exercise, the project consciously sought to make In Control seem interesting, provoking and fun.
- *Make it easy to join in* – Instead of making the pilot special and exclusive, the project was designed as a membership programme for local authorities and entry costs were kept very low. Resources were developed on an open-source basis and shared across the learning community.

This tactic was combined with a constant effort to make the new methodologies really work in practice and to share all the data that was gathered. By 2005, individual budgets were recommended in the Labour Party manifesto and in three government White Papers.

However, political enthusiasm was balanced by scepticism from within academia and the civil service. So this led to the Individual Budget Pilot Programme, which was a government-funded programme to test these ideas in 13 sites across England. It is particularly interesting to note that the combination of political enthusiasm, academic scepticism and civil service resistance to change does not always lead to the design of a rational or enlightening research programme. For instance, the programme was designed to 'test different models of individual budgets' but it actually pooled all the data from each site, making any comparisons impossible.

Furthermore, In Control was to be isolated from the research programme. One senior civil servant instructed In Control to stop using the term 'individual budget' because its term was now a government idea. This meant that In Control had to replace it with 'personal budget' in all its documentation.

Eventually, the continuing political enthusiasm for these ideas overcame the problems within the official research programme, and, in 2007, the government published *Putting People First* (Department of Health, 2007), which declared its intention to extend the use of personal budgets to everyone within social care.

However, policy success is not the same as real changes in people's lives. Today, the implementation of personalisation continues, but there has been little effort to rethink the legal, financial and administrative underpinnings required for successful implementation. Instead, new systems have been bolted onto the old. It is likely that this will lead to a period during which personalisation will officially be declared a success, but where the real impact will be of a much lower quality.

These two stories illustrate a consistent pattern for innovation and resistance to innovation in public services. However, leaders who want to bring about positive change can be mindful of these dynamics in order to understand and minimise the risks faced by any valued change. In summary, we might offer these thoughts:

- The good idea you need is probably being advocated by those who are most dissatisfied with the present set of services. Do you have the capacity to listen and engage with ideas that may seem different?
- New ideas begin to take root when others can join in and try things out for themselves. Do people get the chance to experiment, to connect and to share their learning with each other?
- Policy declarations are not enough. Ideas flourish when older systems are replaced with easier and more effective systems. Do you have the capacity to challenge finance systems, organisational structures or administrative rules?
- Don't 'make people do it' until you are confident that you know how to do it yourself. It is much more important to work with the willing and to define high standards for success than to push for meaningless success too early. Do you have the integrity to seek meaningful change over formal success?

37

From hard to reach to within reach – the 'how' of community engagement in the era of the Big Society

Malik Gul

> We must use the mechanisms of the state to rebuild our societies. (Cameron, 2010)

At a recent meeting of a local public agency, a paper was presented on 'whole system' working. Worryingly, this whole system was only made up of public agencies, hospitals, clinics and GP surgeries, with no mention of the communities and citizens whom they serve or the places in which they congregate and commune. No churches, mosques, temples, gurdwaras, community associations, neighbourhood groups, social networks; nothing at all about the places where people live, work, socialise and play.

These 'associational' places are outside of public agencies and their decision-making processes. They are often grouped together as homogeneous bodies: faith-based organisations, third sector groups, voluntary and community sector organisations, 'charities'. A public agency leader referred to them as a set of random groups that exist outside the professional practice of statutory agencies, as if the only ones who hold a sense of responsibility for the well-being and betterment of our society are the state and its agencies.

Let us examine this randomness. In an inner-city area, there will be Anglican and non-conformist churches, often a growing Pentecostal and black church movement, mosques, temples, and gurdwaras. In Wandsworth, we have approximately 250 faith-based organisations listed, all of whom have influence in their communities far beyond that of any public body. There are also voluntary sector groups, ranging from large ones often patronised by local authorities, through to much smaller ones around black and minority ethnic (BME) communities and refugees and asylum seekers, to even smaller ones like scouts, guides and parents' groups. In Wandsworth, more than 800 voluntary and community sector groups are listed on our database. And this is just 'the known knowns'.

The 'known unknowns' include communities and groups who have yet to find a voice and establish a civic space for themselves, like recently arrived migrants, and non-aligned groups like dominoes clubs, street collectives and self-help groups, all connected with their own members. Alongside these are a whole cadre of community activists, people we call *lightning conductors*: local actors who have credibility and respect within their neighbourhoods.

The English riots of August 2011 showed that there are also 'unknown unknowns': people who don't seem aligned to any recognisable body, yet clearly have grievances to the extent that they participate in socially destructive and criminal activities.

To many, if not most, of these groups, our public agencies are the 'known unknowns'. They exist as symbols of the state, charged with the delivery of our public services. Who are they? How do they make decisions? What resources do they command? Why do they make the choices that they do? How can we influence them? Much of this is lost to the people who these services are intended to serve. They are, often in spite of good intentions, a law and a culture unto themselves, and exist not as part of the community, but in parallel.

Unless we start to develop mechanisms that bring all those who have a concern, interest and responsibility together into dialogue around how our public bodies can work in smarter ways with the systems and infrastructures within our communities, then we will forever be operating partial systems, only ever able to do just about enough for some. The underlying trends writ large in public policy papers – resource reductions, rising demand – will continue to cause a rising tide of health and economic inequalities. This is not good for anybody.

How do we close these gaps and develop processes and systems that deliver services and support in ways that work better for everyone? We are a community empowerment network, independent, community-owned and led. We have acquired a sense of how life is lived underneath the public agency radar and of the potential of everyday people. Let us take local black churches. Some might be a few people meeting regularly, others command the affiliation of hundreds and thousands of people. Our starting point is to figure out who, where and what these nodes of authority and influence are. We have discovered that many prominent community leaders have little knowledge of who their public agencies are and what they do, and no relationship with their fellow leaders who command our public agencies. The best 'outreach' we can expect is that a community development worker, often on the lowest grade, is charged to find out if they can use their church hall to run a health-awareness day!

Yet this church probably commands a weekly attendance of several thousands; even the smallest will have a congregation of several hundreds. And they in turn will be connected with many more through their own neighbourhoods and networks. Which other community leaders have the potential to impact on the behaviours of so many, from BME communities, from poor neighbourhoods – marginalised people who suffer the worst health and social inequalities? The gap between them and public agencies is so great that they are referred to as 'hard to reach', 'seldom heard' or 'difficult to engage'. Yet many community leaders are hearing from and meeting with them daily.

Once we have identified community leaders, and the leaders from public agencies in the parallel universe, the next challenge is to create the spaces in which they can talk and start together to think through ways of working that all can own, embed and sustain. Formal agency meetings just do not do the trick with their formal agenda, sets of papers and set-piece presentations. A lot of meetings in communities are much livelier affairs, people talking over each other, getting up and down to take phone calls and have side conversations, dipping in and out, yet somehow arriving at an agreed end point.

Only by creating spaces where all sides can come together comfortably, where different styles and cultures, languages and narratives can be accommodated and shared, can we begin the co-design journey. We begin to rebuild the trust and confidence that are essential prerequisites for creating better and smarter societies with a sense of shared ownership and responsibility. These conversations need to happen again and again, until we all become good at it. We try to create the enabling world that should sit in the centre of our polity.

From these conversations, shared areas of concern will emerge; a common language and a set of priorities will start to shape and form. Most, if not all, areas of public service delivery meet with concerns community leaders also share. In mental health, we have found common ground. There is gross over-representation of BME communities in in-patient mental health services. An average Trust in-patient service will have around 25% black users from an average population in these communities of about 8%. That over-representation has been the case for several decades, compounded by excessive use of coercive and sectioning practices.

Beginning conversations around these issues has opened up explorations around medicines and diagnostic practices, around statutory powers, around community understanding, and around complex issues of taboo and fear.

Improving Access to Psychological Therapies (IAPT), a national programme designed to deliver talking therapies to those previously unable to access them, enabled us to enter into conversations around mental health and well-being. The local NHS targeted their IAPT services mainly through clinics and GPs. Then they wonder why no one is accessing their services! We have been able to work with community leaders to explain the service and how they can play an active role in its ownership. Following a long period of dialogue, we have started to deliver the services inside community sites. This is not just room hire. The community and its leaders are themselves starting to take ownership over the delivery of services, above and beyond the clinical hours. For example, church sermons on a Sunday are beginning to include the importance of health and well-being as ordered by scripture! This is a journey for both sides. The agencies are not used to allowing community actors to influence their services, to challenge them, to bend the mainstream; and communities are not used to being invited to influence public services. It is by no means perfect or complete but, significantly, we have begun.

In the space of a year, operating out of 10 sites, take-up of IAPT services has increased by 280%, and 580% from BME communities. IAPT is only a start. Mainstream services like diabetes health checks, public health, community safety, all widely needed, all have the potential to be co-produced and delivered in community sites with community leaders acting in ownership roles. The services bring their evidence-based clinical skills and resources, the communities bring their knowledge and reach, and together we design the services in places where people feel comfortable to receive them.

So far, we have established a beachhead. If community-led intelligence and shared dialogues can lead to the co-production of a service like IAPT, imagine what is then possible? We start to use the mechanisms of the state, its statutory powers and resources, to help rebuild our societies, edging towards a radical vision of what a Big Society could be.

38

Disciplined conversation, facilitated dialogue, measured progress

Tim Sims and Fiona Reed

The Prime Minister looked startled and uncomfortable as he cautiously took the offered chair in a circle of 30 NHS doctors, nurses, managers and patients.

It was a morning in September 2007 and, to our surprise, Mr Blair had agreed over breakfast to join our Health Foundation leadership development workshop, being run in the hotel that he was staying in. What made this workshop stand out was patients and users joining NHS 'rising stars', in the role that Bob Sang had christened 'Patient Quality Advisors', to advise on leadership priorities. Tony Blair left his minders at the door and, instead of making a speech to people seated in rows facing him, tentatively sat himself in the circle to join an intriguing dialogue with service users and professionals.

There followed 30 minutes in which we facilitated powerful questions and responses between frustrated patients, weary practitioners and a battered Prime Minister, who that same morning had received a letter from 40 MPs, published in *The Guardian*, demanding his resignation. The conversation encompassed strong emotions, including anger, bafflement and betrayal; shifts in understanding in that room in that short time were palpable. They grew out of a process that acknowledged the emotions without getting stuck in them.

'Discussion' apparently comes from the same somewhat violent and noisy Latin root as concussion and percussion. Facilitating dialogue is more fruitful than trying to facilitate discussion. Facilitating exploration and understanding as a basis for action is at the heart of our work with clinicians, managers and users handling tough dilemmas. It is how we make sure they strengthen their leadership.

That brief encounter, in a focused, facilitated conversation, made an impact on us all. Hours later, Tony Blair opened a widely reported speech on social exclusion to 1,000 people by talking about this unusual dialogue.

Appreciative inquiry

"That conversation on the train was amazing," Mary said with excitement to the others in the leadership development group. Her excitement followed an experimental event designed for the Health Foundation group, in teams with others who they had invited from their own organisations. The process provided guided time, informed by bite-size inputs on organisational culture, for these teams to plan 'culturally savvy' change in their own organisations.

Over sandwiches and crisps on the train journey back from that event, Mary and her colleagues had redesigned a change event for their community matrons scheduled for the following day. Neither matrons nor Mary had been looking forward to it, nervous that the focus would be on what was going badly. Inspired by what they had heard about Appreciative Inquiry, Mary's team decided to focus on what was going well and how the matrons could create more of what worked. The next day, a roomful of sceptical matrons, who initially sat with arms folded, later responded with unexpected willingness. As Mary put it: "Using Appreciative Inquiry like that was definitely a game-changer."

Development time

Much development time in organisations seems to be squandered on bringing people together to listen to 'experts'; facilitating dialogue is about having participants listen to each other. It is about having them exchange and strengthen their own unparalleled expertise on how their organisations work, how best to handle key relationships and how to focus energy on what they determine is really important. Most of all, it is about identifying thoughtful action. Worthy intentions on flipcharts stay that way unless dialogue helps people translate them into intelligent and timely actions.

There are many productive ways that dialogue can be both encouraging and disciplined, leading to the development of thought and to a change in action. This is always our aspiration.

One example was a day-long 'disciplined conversation' between a hundred members of a women's service who had just read a report we had written, which spelled out 18 strong recommendations to improve the service. The discipline was to focus on what they now needed to keep doing, start doing and stop doing, and the planning to make it happen.

Sometimes we work to drive inquiry among clinicians and managers about handling the new leadership structures in which they find themselves. We do this using practical action-learning disciplines, not just to get creative about their huge shared challenges of cost reduction and service improvement, but also to 'get real' about their 80-hour working weeks and the impact these have on their health and the sustainability of their initiatives.

Increasingly, we are coaching small top teams to plan for the important issues that otherwise get submerged in their agenda of urgent ones. We surface assumptions and misunderstandings between them; factors that otherwise may sabotage their commitment to joint actions. We used this process recently with a clinician–manager duo to prevent the failure of their joint commitment to tackling the unhelpful behaviour of some senior doctors. It gave each an opportunity to surface and address some damaging but unstated resentments about apparent breaches of confidentiality. This cleared the way for concerted and thus successful action from them both to build a much stronger professionalism among those doctors.

Time in the turbulent NHS is scarce. In command–and–control environments, time invested in dialogue will be questioned. So those who engage in strong dialogues and disciplined conversations need to demonstrate to themselves and others that they 'work'. For us, that means two things. The first is purpose. We see this simply as increasing the impact of clinicians and managers on the health of their patients and their populations. The second is measurable progress. We help teams identify and score meaningful criteria of success by which they can measure their progress towards the savings, improvements and regulatory standards that their Trusts need to achieve in order to deliver health gains. In our experience, there are few so-called 'soft' factors that cannot be measured against your success criteria. Facilitated dialogue can be and needs to be measured by results.

39

Leadership as if people matter – the Innovative Headteachers Programme

Ian Cunningham

The Innovative Headteachers Programme (IHTP) is one of a number that have brought together six head teachers, with me as a 'learning assistant': assisting the group to function as a context for personal and organisational learning. The programme was run to support innovative heads across the country and was evaluated by the Institute of Education, University of London. Extracts from the full report are reproduced below, including comments of participants.

Self-managed learning

The self-managed learning (SML) approach has been developed over the last 30 years, originally in higher education and with commercial and public sector organisations. In the last 10 years, it has also been used with young people aged 7–16. The approach is more fully described elsewhere (Cunningham, 1999, Cunningham et al, 2000). The IHTP used much the same process as other SML programmes that have catered for senior leaders. However, the focus was on specific issues affecting schools.

The first meeting enabled group members to get to know each other and develop a sound understanding of the process and orientation of the programme. One head teacher's comment that this particular approach "produced increased openness and trust" was strongly endorsed by other group members. In the SML approach, this initial event is crucial in helping senior leaders to create the interpersonal and intellectual basis for effective learning. Without the level of openness and trust that the approach creates, such groups can become more of a talking shop or a short-term problem-solving environment:

> "The exploration of personal issues at the start was crucial."

> "Having a confidential environment is important. The opportunity for heads locally to do this is limited.… It was good to be away from the politics of the city."

> "I can't talk in this deep and open way when I am back in school."

One of the things initiated at the first meeting is a goal-setting process for participants. The structure encourages a strategic focus:

"It's not just about goals: it's also about reflecting on and developing who I am professionally."

"Honing down to a few significant things has been important."

The SML approach distinctively encourages participants to go beyond narrow target-setting and concentrate on big-picture/long-term issues. Also, of particular relevance to the purposes of this programme, participants commented on the importance of exploring values, visions and moral purpose:

"As a result of this programme I have more conversations about moral purpose and values."

"Focus on values and vision has been important for me and for the staff."

"The values of the school have become increasingly important to me."

A place to talk:

"It was better than I expected as local schemes had failed [because] there was too much talk from presenters and not enough space for participants to talk. This approach provided a structure, but it was more open and allowed us to talk."

"The programme gave me a chance to step out of my role and talk openly."

Learning from the SML process

All participants gained new knowledge and skills through the process. However, when asked about significant learning, they focused on other factors. This confirms other research, namely, that in promoting innovation and risk-taking, a knowledge/skills approach is too limited to be of real value. People have to develop in more fundamental ways.

One of these more fundamental ways of promoting innovation and risk-taking concerns the development of self-knowledge and self-awareness. As one participant observed: "The biggest battle has been with myself."

There is a need for those head teachers who are willing to go against the grain or push boundaries to new limits to get a sense that they are doing the right thing educationally, that the risk-taking is responsible, that the taking of a stand is indicative of integrity not intransigence.

"I got affirmation from the group that I was doing the right thing and this helped me in my school. I go for things more whole-heartedly now. I have the courage to be more visible with staff, students and parents and to carry through on ideas."

"The group has given me courage."

"I am braver at tackling the demands of bureaucracy as a result of this group."

Notions like courage take us beyond the realms of efficiency and effectiveness to ambitions and dispositions that have transformational, not merely transactional, intent. In a group of committed, innovative head teachers, this is not altogether surprising. Nor is it surprising to encounter a discourse that acknowledges and affirms the importance of wisdom. Thus, individual heads said of each other:

"You are a wise person. I hope some of the wisdom rubs off on me."

"You know what is important."

"I have been struck by your wisdom."

Unsurprisingly, issues of communication within the contexts of head teachers' daily work constantly surfaced during the course of the programme. One of the outcomes of this recurring preoccupation was the realisation both of the complexity and the necessity of developing deeper understandings of how one does it successfully and that productive communication is more than skills: "I may have felt things were obvious to others, but they were not, so now I communicate better. I tell it straight and avoid others mind-reading."

Clearly, all the participants in the IHTP are significant leaders. However, they talked little about what could be seen as traditional models of leadership. Again, in line with recent developments in the field, where leadership was mentioned, it was often in recognition of how individuals had become more effective systems leaders and had more of a strategic intent, not just strategic plans.

The group unanimously shared the view that: "It was the shared values of the group that helped particularly. This is not something you would get with fellow head teachers within the local authority."

Concluding comments

The responses of the heads to the process in many ways fit with the evidence from other SML programmes for senior leaders (see the references in the box at the end of this chapter). The process of creating a group that provides space for in-depth learning is a powerful approach. The process encourages meta-level ('second-order') learning as participants have to think about what they think about, value what they value, know what they know and how to use it.

Want to know more about self-managed learning?

- Centre for Self Managed Learning website. Available at: www.selfmanagedlearning.org
- Cunningham, I. (1999) *The wisdom of strategic learning*, Aldershot: Gower.
- Cunningham, I., Bennett, B. and Dawes, G. (eds) (2000) *Self-managed learning in action*, Aldershot: Gower.

40

Overview: What kind of leadership?

Jan Walmsley

'Leadership' is a word like 'quality'. It has so many meanings as to be almost useless. And yet, what would we do without it? In one sense, this whole book has been about leadership – many of the authors are leaders; they are at the forefront of implementing change, and taking risks to do so.

We have seen in the academic literature a shift from looking at individual leaders, born not made, to seeking out the secrets of 'leadership', creating systems that operate well without requiring superhuman qualities to glue them together. Peter Drucker put it well:

> No institution can possibly survive if it needs geniuses or supermen to manage it. It must be organised in such a way as to be able to get along under a leadership comprised of ordinary human beings. (Drucker, 1999, p 35)

Today's challenge is to create leadership across as well as within organisations. Since we have yet to get leadership right within discrete organisations, the nature of the challenge is immense.

The authors in this final section have been grappling with what the word 'leadership' means and how it should be exercised if we are to move towards co-production. Undoubtedly, a fluent dialogue across boundaries – which is what we have argued co-produced services require – will demand more inclusive forms of leadership, leadership that is no longer the preserve of the few, but is shared or distributed across organisations and individuals. Change will not happen without different leadership models, although we need to move on from believing, as politicians appear to think, that it is simply a question of putting clinicians rather than managers into positions of power. As Celia Davies puts it in this section:

> To lead change in healthcare is to struggle with the many-headed Hydra that is the NHS.... [I]t ... means more than looking inward. Change-makers at all levels have the task of interpreting the policy regime and delineating, and then monitoring, the space it allows for positive change. They need to be in dialogue with patients and the public – not just explaining change, but giving people the chance to participate in shaping that change. The question is: are our current concepts and understandings of leadership robust enough for the job?

We are not alone in grappling with the question posed here. Warwick Business School academics John Benington and Jean Hartley ask: what would it take to create more effective leadership of the whole governmental and public service system? (Hartley and Benington, 2009, p 3). They say that this question is urgent because recession makes new organisational forms essential, requiring that Holy Grail, a 'whole-systems approach'. They do not have answers; instead, they set out a number of propositions to stimulate debate and they stress '[T]he need for new patterns of "adaptive leadership" to tackle tough complex, cross-cutting problems, where there may be no clear consensus about either the causes or the solutions to the problem' (Hartley and Benington, 2009, p 7).

David Gilbert, one of the authors in this book, frames it differently in another recent publication. His starting point is the importance of valuing the leadership on offer from patients.

> Patients are innovators and entrepreneurs. Ill-health is crisis and opportunity – the crucible within which many have to re-think their lives, reframe and build new identities. Patients and users have the passion and empathy to help others and come up with creative solutions to the difficulties of everyday life. (Gilbert, 2012b, p 2)

Gilbert has also worked on the potential for cost benefits from working with patients (Frontline and InHealth Associates, 2012). His challenges chime with those of systems thinker John Seddon (interviewed in Onyett, 2011), who similarly makes an important connection between taking patients seriously and cost reductions. He believes, and has evidence to demonstrate, that thinking about the service from the perspective of the end user drives out waste and cost. If the person who answers the phone in the call centre, for example, can deal with the caller's issue there and then, enormous savings can be made. It means getting front-line workers to do the job of responding to the customer, rather than referring endlessly up the chain – in effect, to enable them to be leaders.

What these perspectives have in common is the necessity of moving from a provider-dominated system to one where the needs and desires of people who use the system dictate what is provided. This is a big ask, and one that will make considerable demands on our current conceptualisation and practice of leadership.

So the need for fresh thinking is clear, both on what kind of leadership is needed for reinvigorated public services, and on how to develop it. The contributions to this collection do not provide cast-iron answers; rather, they illustrate that the question 'Are our current concepts of leadership robust enough for the job?' is alive and well. In the hunt for fresh thinking, the authors consciously draw on ideas from beyond the health sector – the private sector, community development, education and developments in learning disability over the past 50 years.

The section divides into three parts:

- Reflections on leadership – Two authors reflect on the meanings of leadership with the benefit of hindsight; two practitioners reflect on their own exercise of individual leadership.
- What kind of leadership? – Three chapters seek to envisage the leadership required for co-produced services.
- How to do it? – Two chapters describe approaches to supporting the development of leadership.

Reflections on leadership

The two chapters at the start of this section (Alastair Mant, Celia Davies) use the benefit of hindsight to locate continuities as well as change in leadership. This is important given that the concept of leadership is so 'now'. You would struggle to find the word used in the NHS before 1999. Today, you would struggle to find a policy document, or an inquiry into failings of care or indebted NHS Trusts, which does not use it. We need to be suspicious of the glib response – that faulty leadership is to blame when things go wrong, and that heroic leadership is the reason things go right. As Davies puts it in her chapter, concepts can be used for support rather than illumination. She adds: 'Much talk of leadership, I believe, exhorts more than it illuminates. It directs attention away from some fundamentals.'

So, it is appropriate to open on some pretty solid ground. Despite the superficial attractions of saying everything must change if co-production is to be the order of the day, between them, Davies and Mant remind us of some continuing themes: that good management matters, that it is not a good idea to throw babies out with bathwater. Mant's is a short piece, looking back at fads and trends in 'management'. Appropriately, since so many are entranced by new-style companies, he takes Google's research into its own employees' expectations of a good manager as his exemplar. Maybe it should not come as a surprise that there is continuity between what old-fashioned research tells us about good management and what Google's employees today appear to value:

- Have a clear vision and strategy for the team's work (*My boss is smart*).
- Help your employees with career development (*My boss cares*).
- Do not be a sissy; be productive and results-oriented (*My boss is decisive*).

Above all, says Mant, good bosses keep the important outcomes in mind, they do not attend only to outputs set by targets from elsewhere. Translated into the NHS, this would mean placing patient interests before pleasing politicians and their regulatory proxies. This is far from easy given the pressures to conform but, as the tragedy at Mid Staffordshire NHS Foundation Trust shows (Francis, 2010), overzealous conformity is disastrous leadership, and a tragedy for patients.

Davies uses a long career as a well-informed observer to illustrate the challenges of managing the NHS – challenges that have not gone away just because we try to involve, engage and co-produce. Her 'Hydra' is the uniquely complex matrix of management, medicine and nursing, where all three vie for pre-eminence in determining how the NHS spends its money and organises itself. She helpfully reminds us of the importance of management, and that managers need to face in three directions at once:

- inwards, into the organisations they lead – doing the things Mant described;
- upwards to policy and regulatory directives, to find the spaces these offer for new ideas and approaches (and, I would add, providing an umbrella to protect the employees from the latest fads of politicians where these are not in the best interests of patients); and
- outwards, to engage, involve and inform new constituencies – patients, the public, other organisations.

It is the last of these three that by and large has been the focus of this book, but it is useful to be reminded again of continuities: the medic–versus–manager dance, while nurses – an 'adjunct to a profession' – make do and mend with their yellow stickies. Maybe there is hope that asking all parties to co-design will work, but it is hard to imagine that the embrace can be effective where basic systems and management are so poor.

For Jon Willis, it is quite clear what leadership means. Jon is what is termed in the literature an 'ordinary leader for improvement' (Øvretveit, 2008). His leadership as a ward manager is about recognising that the elderly people in his care are indeed people, and that, despite serious ill-health and dementia, the quality of their lives could be dramatically improved by the deployment of imagination, empathy and some (quite limited) expenditure. To understand his patients' needs, he seeks advice and direction from them, from relatives and from the third sector – he embraces all this in his notion of leadership. The returns are magnificent, not only happier patients, but also active engagement in the life of the ward – 'the pat dog', and the fund-raising for extra support. This is not rocket science. If every ward manager took Jon's approach, would we be hearing the consistent, utterly depressing reports of neglect and poor treatment of elderly people in hospitals? Individuals in front-line management can make a difference. Yet it seems to be so difficult to achieve, and change of this kind is not widespread at present. How can such inspiring leadership be replicated?

There is a parallel here with Kate Hall's message. It is about courage, getting inside the corridors of power and asking down-to-earth questions about quality. The questions are again simple, yet all too often they are not asked. This is seen clearly in spectacular failures of governance across healthcare (Mid Staffordshire) and beyond (Royal Bank of Scotland).

What kind of leadership?

The next three chapters each try to imagine what kind of leadership will be required for the future. Here, it is a matter of putting flesh on the bones. Fine words can inspire but they cannot direct people to action – which is the essence of leadership. The chapter by Nicol and Eaton tries to set out a menu of action for this new type of leadership within the NHS. Simon Duffy and Malik Gul write about leadership within particular communities of practice outside the NHS, and are on the firmer, more concrete ground of practice 'on the ground'.

Ed Nicol and Simon Eaton, young medical consultants, wrestle with what the new professionalism required by co-production will look like. They pick up and run with one of Davies' Hydra heads, the all-important role of doctors, and articulate clearly why change is necessary, referring to those demographic arguments familiar from Wanless (2002) and beyond. It is when they come to describe how the new co-productive leadership will operate that the vision becomes slightly blurred. What they are certain about is that change has to involve a wider community in deciding priorities. We simply cannot go on as we are, with healthcare consuming ever-more resources, and rationing decisions made covertly behind closed doors. They write: 'Crucially, the NHS needs to move from simply collecting feedback to engaging patients and the public in prioritising, designing and delivering improved services.'

They recognise that such an approach requires doctors like them to give up power, while at the same time holding passionately to the value of the trust that the clinician–patient relationship (at its best) can engender. The question is how to hold on to what is best in the classic professional lexicon described by Davies, while at the same time changing the balance of power and the terms of the debate. It is not easy stuff.

The model of 'co-productive health leadership' that they advocate seeks to provide that inclusive map, which aligns clinicians' reflective practice with patients' experiential learning. It may answer Gilbert's question about how to support patient leadership; but will require careful planning and experimentation to get it right.

Simon Duffy looks to leadership lessons from an adjacent sector, learning disability. Services for people with learning disabilities were transformed in the late 20th century, from an almost exclusive reliance on institutions up to the late 1960s, to their discrediting and protracted closure. Leadership for this was threefold, Duffy says:

- passionate thought leadership, provided by the principle of normalisation;
- practical examples of an 'ordinary life' in action, brought together and publicised by the King's Fund; and
- the government falling into line by putting the financial and policy levers in place that eventually resulted in the closure of the last of the large NHS institutions in 2009.

This process was, to an extent, replicated with the introduction of individualised budgets in the early 21st century. The government again belatedly fell into line with the vision of innovators. But Duffy warns of the danger that political attention moves on before improvements are fully embedded, meaning that change can be superficial, and the inherent resistance of large bureaucracies to change can then stall improvement. A related point (on 'mainstreaming' of local initiatives) emerges in the chapter by Jim Phillips in Section 1. Duffy's message is that change comes from leaders outside the system, not from within. He is optimistic overall, although it is important to heed his warnings about the dead hand of government.

Malik Gul provides the final chapter in the 'What kind of leadership?' collection. The experiment he describes was work in progress at the time of publication. He takes communities and their capabilities as his core building block. For him, excellence in public services is about connecting with citizens, drawing, in this case, on the wealth of small- and medium-sized organisations in Wandsworth. His vision is based on practice, his argument is that the initial leadership must come from the statutory sector, reaching out to find and work alongside community leaders so that public agencies move from their parallel existence to being genuinely part of the communities they serve. That way 'hard-to-reach' groups are invited into the conversation, services are redesigned and a start is made in dismantling those startling, apparently intractable, and growing inequalities in health. He ends by citing that elusive 'Big Society'. One could as easily label it as an excellent illustration of leadership working across organisations of different kinds for mutual benefit.

How to do it – where next for leadership development?

The final two chapters take us from what kind of leadership to how it might be encouraged and delivered on the ground.

Tim Sims and Fiona Reed make a case for facilitation as a core practice. If dialogue is to happen across the colliding worlds, then facilitators will be needed to set rules of engagement and make sure that conversations are productive and lead to action, not further disillusionment. They argue for appreciative enquiry: learning from what goes right rather than, as so often happens, from what goes wrong. They propose that quantifiable evidence – that leadership development is effective – is achievable even if it seems elusive.

Finally, Ian Cunningham, bringing ideas from work with leaders in education, develops an important, but often forgotten, theme: leaders do better if their needs as human beings are acknowledged and nurtured. These concerns will be more important than ever as the additional demand of working across localities and services is added to the already prodigious workload piled on organisational leaders. This is a topic also addressed by Rick Stern in Section 2, where, in a counterpoint with Sims and Reed, he addresses the question of what can be done to help leaders face things that, inevitably, do go seriously wrong.

Concluding thoughts

The demands on leadership to create the shift in public services envisioned in this book will be immense. An important question that needs to be addressed is: 'Leadership of what and for what?' Should we be looking at leadership for well-being rather than leadership for and of the NHS? And, if we should, who then are the followers, where does the leader find her constituency? As the situation is so fluid, any distillation of lessons is risky. Tentatively, we propose three:

- Good management still matters – indeed, it matters more, as more people come into the tent, if confusion and disillusionment are not to be the order of the day.
- Space needs to be made for leaders from unexpected quarters – whether they are experts in consumer interfaces, academic advocates or community leaders – who can influence, inspire or partner.
- Those leaders with positions of power inside the system still have an important role: to create the space for experimentation; to go out and connect with the disruptive innovators; and to create the spaces where dialogue across colliding or parallel worlds can happen.

It would be unwise to put too much reliance on leadership, but it would be wise to remember Margaret Mead: 'Never doubt that a small group of committed citizens can change the world. Indeed it is the only thing that ever has' (Mead, no date).

POSTSCRIPT

Better health in harder times – towards a sustainable NHS

As we completed this book, early in 2012, England's NHS was in turmoil. A lengthy and complex Health and Social Care Bill was becoming lengthier, more complex and more contentious in its passage through the legislative process. But the turmoil goes altogether deeper. There is a growing sense that the arrangements we have for public health, public services for healthcare and social care – how as citizens we have access to these and how they relate to each other – are all in need of radical rethinking. More fundamentally still, calls are being made for a new vision to replace the way we live now and the cavalier use that we seem to have made of our shared resources, both human and environmental – in communities, in societies and across the globe. It seems that both our welfare institutions and our wealth-creating institutions are in need of redesign.

The many initiatives described in this book – sometimes small and fragile, yet so often imaginative and energising – suggest that important changes are actually under way. The stories the authors tell are not the isolated incidents that they might look. Over the last few years, there has been a quite remarkable surge of activism and of writing about what is happening with our public services, including health and social care, with myriad case studies showing how things can be different. Born long after the architects of the welfare state, many are reaching towards a more participatory and democratic approach, recognising that a health system has to connect on many levels, and that the public services promise of two generations ago needs to be rethought for the economic and social circumstances of today. Innovations in this area continue apace as we write. For example, the Patient Stories (www.patientstories.org.uk) and Patient Voices (www.patientvoices.org.uk) websites develop and use digital stories to provoke improvement by appealing to the human dimension – in ways also explored by Bacon and Hodgkin in Section 4 of this book.

Apocalyptic predictions about the impossibility of business as usual abound. The Office for Budgetary Responsibility (2011) has warned that the current approach to funding healthcare cannot continue. Costs are expected to rise with an ageing population; the numbers of people with dementia alone are predicted to reach a million in little over a decade. Efficiency gains will help, but it is increasingly being accepted that we need to plan and deliver services in radically different ways. This makes fertile ground for those who call for rationing and the rolling back of the state. But it also opens up the notion of a more sustainable NHS – still supported through tax funding, still available as a right, but more focused on creating health and resilience, and more involving of and accountable to citizens. This theme was opened in Section 1 of this book by Ray Flux, referring to a 'new contract' for health. It links also to the contribution of Nicol and Eaton, for example, seeking a model of leadership that blends sustainability and co-production.

Snapshots of the past

Behind the NHS of 1948 was a powerful unifying vision – a service available across the nation, free at the point of use, with cradle-to-grave entitlement for all secured through insurance. Britain's finest piece of social engineering, born in the solidarity of wartime, was extended into a promise for peace for a population who had lost so much. Politicians of the left and right bought into a wide-ranging state intervention plan for tackling the 'five giants' – want, ignorance, squalor, idleness and disease.

There were compromises from the start. An awkward split between a centralised hospital service, independent GPs and local authority home health and care services was repeatedly tinkered with in successive reforms. Funding prioritised medical innovation and the hospital sector rather than primary care; prevention and promotion of health, not to mention social care, was always the poor relation. Demand increased beyond predictions, investment was limited, covert rationing sometimes had to occur. Renewal of hospital infrastructure was held back, and plans for health centres did not materialise. The health service ran on the commitment of its staff; it was subsidised by a public service ethos of care and by the low pay of many of its employees. Deferential patients did not demur at the wait, and were largely grateful and passive. In practice, healthcare was a profoundly undemocratic experience, sustained by a belief in ever-more wonder drugs and by the advancement of surgical techniques.

The Thatcher era of the 1980s marked a break, although an uneven one. Many insiders were unhappy with the introduction of managerialism, multiple providers and markets. But the NHS was looking decidedly tired, old-fashioned and clunky in what was becoming an increasingly demanding and individualistic culture, with its focus on choice and customer care. Labour in the late 1990s, after a slow start, began to address underinvestment and to introduce rapid-fire service development initiatives from the centre. But its White Paper enshrined much of the neo-liberal critique, with its stress on the need for 'modernisation' (Department of Health, 1997). A great deal was said on paper about patient involvement and citizen participation. In practice, however, it was the shift from 'the patient patient' to the demanding consumer that proceeded apace; and we have some of their voices in Section 4 of this book, for example. Healthcare became about putting ourselves in the ever-more expensive hands of the NHS – a situation that Carle in Section 1 of this book describes as a '20th-century over-professionalisation of care'. The headline issues also remained with the NHS, not with public health and not with social care.

All this enabled analysts to argue that we had to look elsewhere: to the private sector and to countries with mixed models of provision, particularly the US. So, when the credit crunch came, the only answers seemed to be to drive greater efficiency, to shift responsibility to the consumer – making a virtue of choice involving public and private sector options – and paving the way, quite possibly, for the reduction and overt rationing of services. Alternative ideas – refreshing the values of public service and emphasising collective endeavour – needed to emerge.

The challenge of now

Where is the new thinking to be found? There are hints of it in academia, in the traditional political parties and in government publications. But it is in the work of activists on the ground, think-tanks like NEF, NESTA, DEMOS and the RSA, and in web-based discussions and the blogosphere, where new ideas come to life. Think-tank writers have scoured the country to find progressive forms of practice. We use this brief concluding chapter to indicate how the initiatives discussed in the book can be seen as part of a growing social-democratic movement for change. We outline three sets of ideas – at individual, community and societal levels – linking the work of our contributors into progressively wider contexts. First, there is what we call *the power of co-*; second, the renewal of solidarity and community development; and, third, the vision of transition to a more sustainable NHS in a more sustainable society.

The power of co-

The golden thread running through this book has been to demonstrate how much can be achieved when citizens take an active role working in collaboration with service providers, both managing their own care and helping to shape and design services as a whole. Co-production, co-design, co-commissioning – though not necessarily in those words – have been some of the themes contributors have explored.

None of this is entirely new. Promising models emerged in the 1990s, for example, after vigorous campaigning by disabled people's organisations. Individualised or personal budgets began to offer disabled and older people more control over the ways they could spend money allocated to their 'care'. There is a danger, however, in that individualised welfare provision can lead to isolation, and make rationing easier to impose (Morris, 2011). Also, as Duffy observed in Section 5, when governments get their hands on progressive ideas, those ideas can all too easily be corrupted. Creating frameworks for provision with service users collectively is more likely to ensure that the support is available to enable people to control their lives and their choices.

Active involvements such as we have described in this book will not work in all settings and with all groups, but they provide evidence now to show how – with sometimes just a small amount of the right kind of support – expert patients, carers and volunteers can work alongside service providers to create greater well-being and resilience.

Although some dislike the term, *co-production* is the concept that brings together the growing body of work on this theme. A 2009 discussion paper took as its subtitle the proposition that 'transforming health care to involve the public can save money and save lives' (Bunt and Harris, 2009). A little later, an inspiring collection of stories (Boyle et al, 2010) drew on examples from across the UK and internationally to demonstrate how the commitment and creativity of front-line workers, working with those they served, could provide positive outcomes for all. Savings of up to six times the investment in new approaches were estimated. Reading this in parallel with the new material in this book, the report makes for a persuasive story of the power of co-.

If the momentum is to build, ways of *evidencing value* must now be found that are capable of uniting the different stakeholders – funders, front-line workers, politicians, service users and communities. Starts have been made, for example, in the concept of 'social return on investment', in the quest for new outcome-focused methodologies (Substance and NESTA, 2010) and in the arrival of decision tools to help assess and achieve economic benefit from involvement (Frontline and InHealth Associates, 2012). 'Radical efficiency' (Gillinson et al, 2011) – discussed in the overview to the quality section – is relevant here. Transparent accounting for costs will be a key challenge too in the coming years; Foot (Section 3) is one contributor who addresses this directly.

There are objections that must be taken seriously: that changes will effectively mean reductions in funding and service levels, replacing skilled workers with unpaid volunteers, and cutting grants to hard-pressed community providers. Such concerns are very much in the minds of writers discussed above. Authors in this book also underline this. Gul (Section 5) turns cost arguments on their head by arguing for services to 'bend the mainstream', seeking out and working alongside community groups rather than handing responsibilities over to vulnerable and poorly resourced individuals. There is a world of difference between this kind of initiative and approaches that make members of previously disempowered populations into demanding consumers. There is a world of difference, too, between arguing for individual responsibility and activating the power of co-.

Social action and solidarity

If, as some insist, 'people are the principal agents of change in their lives' (Cooke and Gregg, 2010), then people acting in concert in their local communities bring another dimension to what is possible. Community development is a concept that fell out of favour somewhat in the boom years of top-down initiatives in healthy living, economic regeneration and so on. But it is coming back, particularly in the guise of 'asset-based' approaches (see Flux on health promotion in Section 1). Morris and Gilchrist (2011), in a programme of work in this area, emphasise the 'latent resourcefulness' of communities that public policy too often ignores. For them, it is a matter of finding ways to activate social capital through an in-depth understanding of the formal and informal social networks available in particular settings. O'Leary and colleagues (2011) take a wide international sweep, showcasing ways in which rural communities in particular, treating people as their core assets, can be empowered to add value to public services. Foot (2010) embeds the asset approach into health and social care, addressing local councillors, public health specialists and health trust non-executive directors, and indicating ways in which value can be added by working with the assets of a community rather than seeing services as substituting for deficits. Examples are drawn from communities where deprivation and health inequalities are greatest, in the north of England and in London. This analysis neatly contrasts deficit-based thinking, which has characterised so many costly public policy initiatives, with asset-based thinking, which has the potential to do more with less public money. This is also nicely illustrated by Gul's description, in Section 5, of initiatives around mental well-being in Wandsworth.

All this adds a helpful context for some contributions in Section 3, putting more flesh on the concept of collaborative governance. The contributions of Ansell, Keep, Davies and others focus on the dynamics of interaction, stressing the challenges of bringing different worlds together and fostering real dialogue between them. The contributions to Section 4 go on to illustrate the amazing potential, and also some pitfalls, of extending dialogue via new technology.

Whatever the specific forms that organisations may take in the future, it seems certain that the separate worlds of local authorities and the NHS will need to work together ever more closely. Already there is talk of how to encourage elected members to create a co-production vision for their communities, using public health expertise to pull together local intelligence in more creative ways (Solutions for Public Health, 2011). Similarly, while the 'total place' initiative – enabling local authority departments and health service personnel to plan services together – has come to an end, it has sparked a clear, continuing interest in finding ways to foster thinking in the round, and has shown the benefits that can come from taking public service provision out of its silos (Local Government Group, 2011). This is echoed throughout the book, perhaps most directly in Goldberg's chapter in Section 4, which illustrates how local information systems development addressed the issue of NHS silos to achieve both cost and quality goals.

Think – 'sustainable'

If there is one word that brings this thinking together and sets a vision for the renewal of the health system it is 'sustainable'. The Sustainable Development Commission (SDC) was established as an independent agency to advise government back in 2000. Now disbanded, its legacy of ideas and publications is living on and gaining momentum as the economic crisis deepens (www. sd-commissioning.org). At one level, reflecting the history of the concept of sustainability, the SDC's work was concerned with global inequalities and the challenges of international development in the transition to a low carbon future. Underpinning all its work was a growing conviction that we have lost track of what an economy is for. Arguing that economic growth and stability are the means to the end of achieving social and environmental benefits, not ends in themselves, the SDC did much to map out a new kind of economics and delineate a realistic future of 'prosperity without growth'. Some key elements are fewer hours of paid work and more opportunities in the community for using talents to the full, enriching individuals and adding to local resources and capacities.

This is a vision that chimes with calls on the left for a retreat from constant consumption, from defining ourselves by what we have, rather than what we are (Lawson, 2009). It links with the argument that an alternative economic policy needs to get private companies focused on balancing commercial, environmental and social goals (as, for example, in the notion of integrated reporting, mentioned at the end of Section 2). And it offers a future beyond austerity alone (see, eg, Smith and Bozier, 2011). The 'great transition' programme of the New Economics Foundation takes this perhaps furthest in its focus on the 'core economy' – the resources embedded in everyday life – and in its aim to move from 'an economy based on scarcity of economic resources to one based on an abundance of human resources' (Coote, 2011, p 4).

The clearest illustration of this approach in this book is the work around community champions described by Furr in Section 3. We could go further, however, in looking to the potential of the NHS to foster new ways of working in social enterprises and mutuals (http://healthandcare.dh.gov.uk/r2p-case-studies). Procurement also offers potential. Some NHS bodies have signed up to be good corporate citizens in procurement (www.corporatecitizen.nhs.uk), and they offer case studies to demonstrate how using local enterprise can add to the wider social, environmental and economic vibrancy of a local area. An NHS Sustainable Development Unit is also in action (www.sdu.nhs.uk). A report early in 2012 summarised progress, covering the views of NHS leaders and demonstrating public support for these issues (NHS Sustainable Development Unit, 2012).

Not surviving, but thriving

What, finally, does this new writing and activism amount to? Are we moving from welfare to well-being – from an *entitlements* frame of mind that is essentially passive, to an *engagement* one, supporting the parts that people can play in developing their own well-being and that of others, through shared decision-making and active citizenship? Both our contributors and the writers discussed here would seem to suggest that the answer can be 'yes'. The stories they tell and the concepts that they use are not about *surviving* in the era of austerity in which we find ourselves, they are about *thriving* in it. Better health in harder times can be much more than a slogan. And this brings us back to the man who was the inspiration for this book. In an inaugural lecture given in 2007, Bob Sang was talking of a sustainable NHS, and arguing that engagement and involvement were core business for the NHS (see Sang and Cowper, 2010). As he so often said, 'over to you'.

References

Abelson, J., Forest, P.-G., Eyles, J., Smith, P., Martin, E. and Gauvin, F.-P. (2002) 'Obtaining public input for health-system decision-making – past experiences and future prospects', *Canadian Public Administration*, vol 45, no 1, pp 70–97.

Aked, J., Marks, N., Cordon, C. and Thompson, S. (2008) *Five ways to wellbeing – a report presented to the Foresight Project on communicating the evidence base for improving people's wellbeing*, London: New Economics Foundation. Available at: www.neweconomics.org/publications/five-ways-well-being-evidence

Ansell, C. and Gash, A. (2008) 'Collaborative governance in theory and practice', *Journal of Public Administration Research and Theory*, vol 18, no 4, pp 543–71.

Barnes, M. (2008) 'Passionate participants – emotional experiences and expressions in deliberative forums', *Critical Social Policy*, vol 28, pp 461–81.

Barnes, M., Skelcher, C., Beirens, H., Dalziel, R., Jeffares, S. and Wilson, L. (2008) *Designing citizen-centred governance*, Birmingham: University of Birmingham/ Joseph Rowntree Foundation. Available at: www.jrf.org.uk/publications/ designing-citizen-centred-governance

Bate, S.P. and Robert, G. (2007) *Bringing user experience to health care improvement – the concepts, methods and practices of experience-based design*, Oxford: Radcliffe Publishing.

Bechel, D., Myers, W. and Smith, D.G. (2000) 'Does patient centred care pay off?', *Joint Commission Journal of Quality Improvement*, vol 26, no 7, pp 400–9.

Blaffer Hrdy, S. (2009) *Mothers and others – the evolutionary origins of mutual understanding*, Cambridge: Harvard University Press.

Boyce, T., Dixon, A., Fasolo, B. and Reutskaja, E. (2010) *Choosing a high-quality hospital – the role of nudges, scorecard design and information*, London: The King's Fund.

Boyle, D. and Harris, M. (2011) *The challenge of coproduction*, London: NESTA.

Boyle, D., Slay, J. and Stephens, L. (2010) *Public services inside out – putting coproduction into practice*, London: NESTA/NEF/The Lab. Available at: www.nesta.org.uk/ publications/reports/assets/features/public_services_inside_out

Brewis, R. and Fitzgerald, J. (2011) *Citizenship in health*, Sheffield: In Control.

Bullivant, J. and Corbett-Nolan, A. (2011) 'The King III – a model of governance for the new NHS? Briefing note prepared for Prof. Mervyn King's NHS London lecture, 29 Nov 2011'. Available at: good-governance.org.uk/Product%20 Menus/king-iii-report-briefing-note.htm

Bunt, L. and Harris, M. (2009) *The human factor – how transforming healthcare to involve the public can save money and save lives*, London: NESTA/The Lab. Available at: www.nesta.org.uk/library/documents/the-human-factor.pdf

Cabinet Office (2011) 'Open data measures in the Autumn Statement'. Available at: www.cabinetoffice.gov.uk/news/open-data-measures-autumn-statement

Cameron, D. (2010) 'Big society', Hugo Young lecture. Available at: www. guardian.co.uk/politics/video/

Chapman, R. and Lowndes, V. (2009) 'Accountable, authorized or authentic? What do "faith representatives" offer urban governance?', *Public Money and Management*, November, pp 371–8.

Cheshire, A. and Ridge, D.T. (2012) 'Evaluation of the experience led commissioning in end of life care project'. Available at: http://westminsterresearch.wmin. ac.uk/10257/

Chief Medical Officer (2009) Personal communication.

Clarke, J. and Newman, J. (1997) *The managerial state*, London: Sage.

Colin-Thomé, D. (2009) *A review of lessons learned for commissioners and performance managers following the Healthcare Commission investigation*, London: Mid Staffordshire NHS Foundation Trust.

Conservative Party (2010) *Invitation to join the government of Britain – general election manifesto 2010*, London: The Conservative Party.

Cooke, G. and Gregg, P. (eds) (2010) *Liberation welfare*, London: DEMOS. Available at: www.demos.co.uk/publications/liberationwelfare

Coote, A., with Goodwin, N. (2011) *The great transition – social justice and the core economy. Working paper 1*, London: NEF.

Cowper, A., Keep, J. and Sang, B. (2004) 'Opening our eyes to choice, risk and accountability', *British Journal of Healthcare Management*, vol 10, no 11, pp 329–33.

Cunningham, I. (1999) *The wisdom of strategic learning*, Aldershot: Gower.

Cunningham, I., Bennett, B. and Dawes, G. (eds) (2000) *Self-managed learning in action*, Aldershot: Gower.

Davies, C. (1995) *Gender and the professional predicament in nursing*, Buckingham: Open University Press.

Davies, C. (2003) 'Workers, professions and identity', in Henderson, J. and Atkinson, D. (eds) *Managing care in context*, London: Routledge.

Davies, C., Wetherall, M. and Barnett, E. (2006) *Citizens at the centre – deliberative participation in healthcare decisions*, Bristol: The Policy Press.

Department of Health (1997) *The new NHS – modern, dependable*, Cm 3807, London: The Stationery Office.

Department of Health (1999) *Saving lives: our healthier nation*, Cm 4386, London: The Stationery Office.

Department of Health (2001) *The expert patient: a new approach to chronic disease management for the 21st century*, London: The Stationery Office.

Department of Health (2006) *Our health, our care, our say: a new direction for community services*, London: The Stationery Office.

Department of Health (2007) *Putting people first: a shared vision and commitment to the transformation of adult social care*, London: The Stationery Office.

Department of Health (2008) *High quality care for all – NHS next stage review, final report (Darzi report)*, Cm 7432, London: The Stationery Office.

Department of Health (2009) 'Guidance on direct payments for community care, services for carers and children's services – England 2009'. Available at: www.dh.gov. uk/en/Publicationsandstatistics/Publications/PublicationsPolicyAndGuidance/ DH_104840

Department of Health (2010a) *Equity and excellence – liberating the NHS*, Cm7881 (Gateway 14385), London: The Stationery Office.

Department of Health (2010b) 'Quality accounts provider survey'. Available at: www.dh.gov.uk/prod_consum_dh/groups/dh_digitalassets/@dh/@en/documents/digitalasset/dh_122542.pdf

Department of Health (2010c) *National Quality Board – Annual report 2009/10*, London: Department of Health.

Department of Health (2010d) *An information revolution: a consultation on proposals*. Available at: www.dh.gov.uk/en/Consultations/Liveconsultations/DH_120080

Department of Health (2011) 'Quality, Innovation, Productivity and Prevention (QIPP)'. Available at: www.dh.gov.uk/en/Healthcare/Qualityandproductivity/QIPP

Department of Health (2012) 'Update on personal health budgets March 2012'. Available at: www.dh.gov.uk/health/files/2012/03/Personal-Health-Budget-newsletter-March-2012.pdf

Dias, J., Eardley, M., Harkness, E., Townson, L., Brownlee-Chapman, C. and Chapman, R. (2012) 'Keeping wartime memory alive – an oral history project about people with learning difficulties in Cumbria', *Disability and Society*, vol 27, no 1, pp 31–49.

Docherty, A., Harkness, E., Eardley, M., Townson, L. and Chapman, R. (2006) 'What they want, yes! But what we want; bugger us!', in Mitchell, D., Traustadottir, R., Chapman, R., Townson, L., Ingham, N. and Ledger, S. (eds) *Exploring experiences of advocacy by people with learning disabilities*, London: Jessica Kingsley.

Drucker, P. (1999) *Management challenges for the 21st century*, New York, NY: Harper Collins.

Eardley, M. (2001) 'The way of life', unpublished manuscript.

Equality and Human Rights Commission (2011) 'Close to home – an inquiry into older people and human rights in home care'. Available at: www.equalityhumanrights.com

Foot, C. and Ross, S. (2010) *Accounting for quality to the local community – findings from focus group research*, London: The King's Fund.

Foot, C., Raleigh, V., Ross, S. and Lyscom, T. (2011) *How do quality accounts measure up? Findings from the first year*, London: The King's Fund.

Foot, J., with Hopkins, T. (2010) *A glass half full – how an asset approach can improve community health and wellbeing*, London: Improvement and Development Agency. Available at: www.idea.gov.uk/idk/aio/18410498

Francis, R. (2010) *Independent inquiry into care provided by Mid Staffordshire NHS Foundation Trust, January 2005–March 2009, vol 1* (HC375-I), London: The Stationery Office.

Freidson, E. (1970) *Profession of medicine – a study of the sociology of applied knowledge*, New York, NY: Dodd, Mead.

Frontline and InHealth Associates (2012) 'The economic case for involvement'. Available at: www.inhealthassociates.co.uk/index.php/articles/

Fung, C., Lim, Y.-W., Mattke, S., Danberg, C. and Shekelle, P.G. (2008) 'Systematic review – the evidence that publishing patient care performance data improves quality of care', *Annals of Internal Medicine*, vol 148, no 2, pp 111–23.

Garcia-Alamino, J.M., Ward, A.M., Alonso-Coello, P., Perera, R., Bankhead, C., Fitzmaurice, D. and Heneghan, C.J. (2010) 'Self-monitoring and self-management of oral anticoagulation', *Cochrane Database of Systematic Reviews*, vol 4 (Art No CD003839): DOI: 10.1002/14651858.CD003839.pub2.

Gauvin, F.-P., Abelson, J., Giacomini, M., Eyles, J. and Lavis, J.N. (2010) '"It all depends" – conceptualising public involvement in the context of health technology assessment agencies', *Social Science and Medicine*, vol 70, pp 1518–76.

Gilbert, D. (2012a) 'Empowering the new generation of patient leaders'. Available at: www.inhealthassociates.co.uk/index.php/articles/

Gilbert, D. (2012b) 'The rise of the patient leader', *Health Service Journal*, January. Available at: www.inhealthassociates.co.uk/index.php/articles/

Gillinson, S., Horne, M. and Baeck, P. (2011) *Radical efficiency – different, better, lower cost public services*, London: NESTA. Available at: www.nesta.org.uk/publications/assets/features/radical_efficiency

Goffman, E. (1968) *Stigma – notes on the management of a spoiled identity*, Harmondsworth: Penguin.

Griffiths Report (1983) *NHS management inquiry*, London: Department of Health and Social Security.

Greenhalgh, T., Humphrey, C. and Woodard, F. (eds) (2010) *User involvement in health care*, New Jersey, NJ: Wiley-Blackwell.

Hackney LINk (2011) 'Rate our service – Hackney'. Available at: www.rateourservice.co.uk/hackney

Harrison, S. and Lim, J.N.W. (2003) 'The frontier of control – doctors and managers in the NHS 1966 to 1997', *Clinical Governance*, vol 8, no 1, pp 13–18.

Hartley, J. and Benington, J. (2009) *Whole systems go! Improving leadership across the whole public service system – propositions to stimulate discussion and reform*, Ascot: Sunningdale Institute National School of Government.

Health Foundation (2011) *Helping people help themselves*, London: Health Foundation.

HQIP (Health Quality Improvement Partnership) (2011) 'National adult cardiac surgical database (Healthcare Quality Improvement Partnership)'. Available at: www.hqip.org.uk/national-adult-cardiac-surgical-database

Hunt, P. (ed) (1966) *Stigma – the experience of disability*, London: Chapman.

Iles, V. (2011) 'Why reforming the NHS doesn't work – the importance of understanding how good people offer bad care'. Available at: www.reallylearning.com (also available from Amazon and www.lulu.com).

iWantGreatCare (2011) 'iWantGreatCare'. Available at: www.iwantgreatcare.com

Keep, J. (2007) 'Making an impact through integrating learning methodologies – a large scale, collaborative, systems-based learning network in the British National Health Service', in S. Sambrook and J. Stewart (eds) *Human resource development in the public sector – the case of health and social care*, London: Routledge.

Keep, J. and Sang, B. (2005) 'Engaging the intermediate tier in "a patient-led NHS"', *British Journal of Healthcare Management*, vol 11, no 7, pp 204–8.

Kennedy, R. and Phillips, J. (2010) 'Social return on Investment (SROI) – a case study with an expert patient programme', *SelfCare*, vol 2, no 1 pp 10–20. Available at: www.selfcarejournal.com/view.abstract.php?id=10035

King's Fund (2011) *The future of leadership and management in the NHS – no more heroes*, London: The King's Fund.

Lawson, N. (2009) *All consuming – how shopping got us into this mess and how we can find our way out*, London: Penguin.

Learmonth, M., Martin, G.P. and Warwick, P. (2009) 'Ordinary and effective – the catch-22 in managing the public voice in health care?', *Health Expectations*, vol 12, pp 106–15.

Litva A., Canvin, K., Shepherd, M., Jacoby, A. and Gabbay, M. (2009) 'Lay perceptions of the desired role and type of user involvement in clinical governance', *Health Expectations*, vol 12, no 1, pp 81–91.

Local Government Group (2011) *Productive places – continuing the focus on place based improvement*, London: Local Government Improvement and Development. Available at: www.local.gov.uk

Marx, K. (1867) *Capital*, vol 1, Moscow: Progress Publishers.

May, J. (2007) 'The triangle of engagement – an unusual way of looking at the usual suspects', *Public Money and Management*, February, pp 69–75.

Mead, M. (no date). Available at: www.leadershipnow.com/leadershipquotes.html

Morris, D. and Gilchrist, A. (2011) *Communities connected – inclusion, participation and common purpose*, London: RSA. Available at: www.thersa.org/__data/assets/pdf_file/0011/518924/RSA_Communities-Connected-AW_181011.pdf

Morris, J. (1993) *Independent lives – community care and disabled people*, Basingstoke: MacMillan.

Morris, J. (2011) *Rethinking disability policy*, York: Joseph Rowntree Foundation. Available at: www.jrf.org.uk/sites/files/jrf/disability-policy-equality-summary.pdf

NHS London (2011) 'GP outcome standards'. Available at: www.myhealth.london.nhs.uk/outcome-standards

NHS Sustainable Development Unit (2012) 'Sustainability in the NHS – health check 2012'. Available at: www.sdu.nhs.uk/publications-resources/89/sustainability-in-the-nhs-health-check-2012/

NHS West Midlands (2008) *Long term conditions clinical pathway report*, Birmingham: NHS West Midlands.

Nicol, E. and Sang, B. (2010) 'A coproductive health leadership model to support the liberation of the NHS', *Journal of the Royal Society of Medicine*, vol 104, pp 64–8.

North West SHA (2007) 'Patient opinion – roll out across the Northwest'. Available at: www.northwest.nhs.uk/document_uploads/Board_Papers/08.PatientOpinion.pdf

Nyadzayoo, M. (2011) 'In praise of managers', *Health and Care Weekly*, 8 (November).

Office for Budgetary Responsibility (2011) *Economic and fiscal outlook*, Cm 8218, London: The Stationery Office.

O'Leary, T., Braithwaite, K. and Burkett, I. (2011) *Appreciating assets – report from the International Association for Community Development (IACD)*, Dunfermline: Carnegie United Kingdom Trust. Available at: www.iacdglobal.org/publications-and-resources/IACD-publications

Onyett, S. (2011) 'Interview with John Seddon', *International Journal of Leadership in Public Services*, vol 7, no 1, pp 62–7.

Øvretveit, J. (2008) 'Leading improvement effectively', *The Health Foundation*. Available at: www.health.org.uk/publications/leading-improvement-effectively/

Parsons, T. (1975) 'The sick role and the role of the physician reconsidered', *Milbank Memorial Fund Quarterly*, vol 53, no 5, pp 257–78.

Patient Opinion (2011) 'Patient opinion'. Available at: www.patientopinion.org.uk

Patients' Association (2011a) 'We've been listening – have you been learning?'. Available at: www.patients-association.com/Portals/0/Public/Files/Research%20Publications/We%27ve%20been%20listening,%20have%20you%20been%20learning.pdf

Patients' Association (2011b) 'Patients Association launches damning report into poor care in England's Hospitals', press release, 9 November. Available at: www.patients-association.com/Default.aspx?tabid=81&Id=23

Porter, R. (1997) *The greatest benefit to mankind – a medical history of humanity from antiquity to the present*, London: Harper Collins.

Sanderson, H., Kennedy, J., Ritchie, P. and Goodwin, G. (1997) *People, plans and possibilities – exploring person centred planning*, Edinburgh: Scottish Human Services.

Sang, B. (2002) 'Modernising patient and public involvement in health', *British Journal of Healthcare Management*, vol 8, no 10, pp 380–5.

Sang, B. (2007) 'A citizen-led coalition for integrated care', *Journal of Integrated Care*, vol 15, no 3, pp 44-52.

Sang, B. (2009) 'Health gain – the true test of quality for 21st century healthcare', *Health Policy Insight*, vol 6 (September). Available at: www.healthpolicyinsight.com/?q=node/304

Sang, B. and Cowper, A. (2010) 'Whose healthcare business is it anyway?', Inaugural lecture, *British Journal of Healthcare Management*, London South Bank University.

Shirky, C. (2008) *Here comes everybody – the power of organizing without organizations*, Harmondsworth: Penguin, Allen Lane.

Smith, A. and Bozier, L. (2011) 'Labour's business – why enterprise must be at the heart of Labour politics in the 21st century'. Available at: www.laboursbusiness.org.uk

Social Innovation eXchange (2008) 'Patient Opinion – case study by School for Social Entrepreneurs'. Available at: www.socialinnovationexchange.org/ideas-and-inspiration/health-and-wellbeing/case-study/patient-opinion

Solutions for Public Health (2011) *Coproduction for health – a new model for a radically new world. Building new approaches to delivery to achieve better health outcomes at the local level. Final report of a national colloquium Dec 2011*, Oxford: Solutions for Public Health. Available at: www.sph.nhs.uk/lgcolloquiumreport

Spedding, F., Harkness, E., Townson, L., Docherty, A., McNulty, N. and Chapman, R. (2002) 'The role of self advocacy – stories from a self advocacy group from the experiences of its members', in B. Gray and R. Jackson (eds) *Advocacy and learning disability*, London: Jessica Kingsley.

Stewart, J. (1996) 'Innovation in democratic practice in local government', *Policy & Politics*, vol 24, no 1, pp 29–41.

Storey, J., Bullivant, J. and Corbett-Nolan, A. (2011) *Governing the new NHS – issues and tensions in health service management*, London: Routledge.

Strathern, M. (2000) *Audit cultures – anthropological studies in accountability, ethics and the academy*, London: Routledge.

Strauss, A. and Glaser, B. (1975) *Chronic illness and the quality of life*, St Louis, MO: Mosby.

Substance and NESTA (National Endowment for Science, Technology and the Arts) (2010) *Whose story is it anyway? Evidencing impact and value for better public services*, London: NESTA. Available at: www.nesta.org.uk/publications/assets/features/whose_story_is_it_anyway

Swain, J. and French, S. (2000) 'Towards an affirmation model of disability', *Disability & Society*, vol 15, no 4, pp 569–82.

Thomas, C. (2007) *Sociologies of disability and illness*, Basingstoke: Palgrave MacMillan.

Towell, D. (1988) *An ordinary life in practice – developing comprehensive community based services for people with learning disabilities*, London: King Edward's Hospital Fund for London.

Townson, L. (2004) 'There is no such word as can't!', unpublished manuscript.

Townson, L., Macauley, S., Harkness, E., Docherty, A., Dias, J., Eardley, M. and Chapman, R. (2007) 'Research project on advocacy and autism', *Disability & Society*, vol 22, no 5, pp 523–36.

UPIAS (Union of the Physically Impaired against Segregation) and TDA (The Disability Alliance) (1976) *Fundamental principles of disability*, London: UPIAS.

Wanless, D. (2002) *Securing our future health – taking a long-term view*, London: Public Enquiry Unit, HM Treasury.

Wanless, D. (2004) *Securing good health for the whole population: final report*, London: The Stationery Office.

West, L. (2004) 'Doctors on the edge – a cultural psychology of learning and health', in P. Chamberlayne, J. Bornat and U. Apitzsch (eds) *Biographical methods and professional practice*, Bristol: The Policy Press.

Year of Care (2011a) 'Working together for better healthcare and better self care – Year of Care Programme'. Available at: www.diabetes.nhs.uk/year_of_care

Year of Care (2011b) 'Thanks for the Petunias – a guide to developing and commissioning non-traditional providers to support the self-management of people with long term conditions'. Available at: www.diabetes.nhs.uk/year_of_care

Index